Interprofessional Perspectives of Mental Health Crisis

Interprofessional Perspectives of Mental Health Crisis

For nursing, health, and the helping professions

Edited by Kris Deering and Jo Williams

Open University Press

Open University Press
McGraw Hill
8th Floor, 338 Euston Road
London
England
NW1 3BH

email: enquiries@openup.co.uk
world wide web: www.openup.co.uk

and Two Penn Plaza, New York, NY 10121-2289, USA

First published in this edition 2022

A catalogue record of this book is available from the British Library

ISBN-13: 9780335250493
ISBN-10: 0335250491
eISBN: 9780335250509

Library of Congress Cataloging-in-Publication Data
CIP data applied for

Typeset by Transforma Pvt. Ltd., Chennai, India

Praise page

"This publication is a valuable and timely resource given the increasing recognition of the impact of mental health needs in a range of different professional settings. The variety of professional contributions in each chapter helps to foster a culture of mutual understanding of the roles and challenges for different professionals when supporting someone experiencing a mental health crisis. By sharing their knowledge and experiences, the diverse range of professionals involved in this book seek to bring about improved collaborative working, and ultimately more positive outcomes for all involved."

Victoria Sweetmore, University of Derby

"Any one of us could experience a mental health crisis. However, a high-quality interdisciplinary response can be lifesaving and life changing.

This book is an important contribution to the literature as it has examples of good practice for all professionals – both on the frontline and in service development.

It has advice on maintaining compassionate care in what can be incredibly demanding situations and looks at ways to keep mental health services at the centre of emergency and crisis response. It has practical steps to safeguard against the challenges of fragmentation, diffusion of responsibility and limited resources. Crucially, at its heart, there is an emphasis on integration and collaboration with patients and carers."

Dr Adrian James, President, Royal College of Psychiatrists

"Mental health crisis care is a complex area, which deserves a highly skilled response. It is vital for all agencies involved to collaborate alongside mental health services. This book has something for everyone: each chapter offers advice that will enhance the practice of a different professional group and will give others insight into other perspectives. It contains a blueprint for improving care, from practical advice for frontline response, to policy aspects needed for service integration. Above all it emphasises the pivotal role of liaison psychiatry for patients in acute hospitals, and crisis resolution home treatment teams in the community, and the importance of learning from lived experience of crisis care."

Dr Annabel Price, Chair, Faculty of Liaison Psychiatry, Royal College of Psychiatrists

Contents

Contributors

Kris Deering is a Senior Lecturer in Mental Health Nursing at the University of the West of England, Bristol. He is the Module Lead of working with a person experiencing a mental health crisis, which was the inspiration for this text. Kris has experience as a Senior Nurse Practitioner leading clinical care within a Crisis Resolution Home Treatment team and is also involved with developing risk management within acute mental healthcare to integrate patient recovery within its practices, the topic of his PhD study. Kris has a keen interest in the philosophies underpinning mental healthcare, looking at tangible ways to promote the service user's voice to ensure that care is person-centred.

Anne Eason is Acting Associate Head of Department (Policing) and a Senior Lecturer at the University of the West of England, Bristol, working collaboratively with Avon and Somerset Police. Formerly a Senior Probation Officer, Anne combines her operational experience with her academic knowledge in the teaching of policing programmes and has a particular interest in the influence of emotional intelligence in police decision making, especially in relation to domestic and sexual violence. Anne is actively involved in police-related research and the pedagogical experiences of officers in the professionalisation process.

Matt Gaunt is a Senior Lecturer in Policing at the University of the West of England, Bristol. Matt is the Programme Leader for the Degree-Holder Entry Programme in Policing, which develops the next generation of detectives for Avon and Somerset Constabulary. As a former police officer, Matt has significant professional experience with those in mental health crisis, as well as an academic interest in the treatment of suspects with complex needs in the criminal justice system.

Andy Hill is a Clinical Nurse Specialist, Liaison Psychiatry, at Bristol Royal Infirmary. Andy has 37 years of clinical experience in a range of settings, including acute inpatient, forensic, drug and alcohol, and community mental health. For the last eight years, Andy has combined clinical work in liaison psychiatry with an Associate Lecturer role at the University of the West of England, Bristol. He has a particular interest in the interface between philosophy and mental health, including the ethical issues relating to suicide.

Jordan Hodge is a Service Manager for the Bristol Crisis Service, Avon and Wiltshire Mental Health Partnership (NHS) and an Associate Lecturer in Mental Health at the University of the West of England, Bristol. He previously worked in psychiatric intensive inpatient care (PICU) and community mental health crisis services. Jordan also has a keen interest in pharmacology and medication management and has held various roles as a Lead Prescriber and Clinical Nurse Specialist. In his Associate Lecturer role at UWE, Jordan works with pre- and post-registration students, including in nursing and paramedic science.

Robert Lomax is a Senior Lecturer in Social Work at the University of the West of England, Bristol. Robert is also a registered social worker, a former senior practitioner and qualified approved mental health professional (AMHP). He is a Thorn-trained practitioner in integrated approaches to psychosocial interventions in mental healthcare. He worked for The Open University (2008–2017) and has been at the University of the West of England since 2017. He is the Programme Leader for UWE's AMHP training programme. Robert is also undertaking doctoral research exploring how social workers use their knowledge of the social determinants of mental health to inform their practice.

Amy Manley is a Consultant Liaison Psychiatrist at University Hospitals Bristol NHS Foundation Trust. She leads on the psychiatric care of inpatients and people attending the emergency department of an acute hospital. She has recently been appointed as the Lead for Undergraduate Psychiatry Teaching at the University of Bristol Medical School. Prior to commencing her PhD at the University of Bristol, she worked there as a Teaching Unit Developer on the Teaching and Learning for healthcare professionals Master's Degree course. Her research interests are in the fields of liaison psychiatry and medical education with a particular interest in student mental health.

Stevie Morris is Student Placement Lead for Devon Partnership Trust, having previously worked in a range of services, including CAMHS, Assertive Outreach and Older Adult care. While a student nurse at the University of the West of England, Stevie developed a model for group supervision; this was designed for students and newly qualified nurses, with interprofessional transferability. Work on the PIPS (Peer Inter-Professional Supervision) model has won several conference awards and is being embedded into preceptorship training across the South West of England. Stevie continues to engage in pre- and post-registration nurse education and training.

Rob Starr is a Senior Lecturer in Policing at the University of the West of England, Bristol, working on the Police Constable Degree Apprenticeship programme. Prior to joining the teaching team at UWE, Rob had been a police officer for 28 years, beginning in the Metropolitan Police before transferring to the West Midlands Police. Rob has a wide variety of experience within operational law enforcement, both as a uniformed officer and as a detective, which he is actively building upon in academic research. Currently Rob is developing research projects into policing responses to mental health and possible precursor factors apparent in terrorist radicalisation.

Kevin Stone is an Associate Professor in Social Work at the University of Plymouth. He is also a registered social worker, a practising approved mental health professional (AMHP) and qualified Best Interest Assessor. Dr Stone is an active researcher in the field of mental health law and health and social care practice and, as an author, has published widely. He has been a social work academic for over 10 years, teaching health and social care law, social work skills and social sciences. Dr Stone was formerly the programme leader for the AMHP programme and latterly an Associate Head of Department for Law at the University of the West of England, Bristol.

David Williams is a Senior Lecturer in Paramedic Science at the University of the West of England, Bristol. He has a keen academic interest in mental capacity and mental health legislation, specifically around the application by emergency responders. David still practises clinically as a paramedic within the Bristol region.

Jo Williams is a Senior Lecturer in Mental Health Nursing at the University of the West of England, Bristol. Jo is a registered mental health nurse and joined UWE in 2010. She has worked in both military and civilian healthcare settings and as a clinical nurse specialist, supporting people living with co-existing mental health and substance use issues. Dr. Williams has a keen interest in promoting interprofessional working and is currently engaged in research exploring the lived experience of social media influencers and their mental health and well-being.

Rob Williams is a Senior Lecturer in Mental Health Nursing at the University of the West of England, Bristol. Rob has worked across several programmes, including undergraduate (BSc Mental Health nursing) and postgraduate (independent prescribing and medication management) studies. He is a registered mental health nurse, independent prescriber and dialectical behaviour therapist with a keen interest in pharmacology, medication management and crisis/acute care. Between 2009 and 2012, Rob worked as a newly qualified nurse and then as a charge nurse in psychiatric intensive care (PICU) before taking several roles with prison psychiatry between 2012 and 2018, which included: senior mental health practitioner, Team Lead for mental health and substance misuse services and Clinical lead for prescribing across two prisons in the South West of England.

Foreword

When I picked up this book, I thought about what I hoped to find. What would be important and useful for a health or social care student or practitioner to learn and understand when thinking about supporting people in a mental health crisis?

My first thought concerned the experiences and perspectives of service users and their families or carers. In my first job as a mental health nurse, working in a mental health day centre, I attended a talk given by Louise Pembroke, a young service user activist who spoke passionately about the appalling treatment being experienced by people in mental health crises who self-harmed and had contact with the health services, such as ambulance staff and medics and nurses in emergency departments. As a young newly qualified nurse, I was both unnerved by the anger and challenge that Louise understandably displayed towards healthcare professionals and upset by the stories of stigmatising language, cruel indifference and much worse experienced by people already in severe anguish. Now, many years later as a Professor of Mental Health Nursing, I work alongside researchers, clinicians and people with lived experience of self-harm and suicidal intent, to investigate how we can improve the care and treatment received by people in similar mental health crises when they arrive at an emergency department.

The chapters of this book very much engage with those experiences and provide humane, empathic, skilled, therapeutic approaches for those looking to understand how to better engage, care for and work alongside those in such depths of despair and, hopefully, to collaboratively find a way forward.

My second thought, as a researcher, was whether this book drew on relevant research evidence to inform the reader and support the arguments and recommendations being made. It was pleasing to see chapters well supported by up-to-date evidence and key seminal texts that remain important. In addition, the author of each chapter has provided suggestions for further reading and I've already dipped into a few of those.

My third thought concerned interprofessional working and learning. One of my earlier clinical roles was as a community mental health nurse, working with people who were homeless, mentally ill, and very often using alcohol and other substances. As part of a small inter-agency team, I was soon learning the crucial importance and also major challenges of working with and alongside a range of healthcare providers, social workers, drug and alcohol workers, police and probation services, housing officers and agencies, and most especially a vast range of voluntary and faith organisations that were often leading the way in trying to engage with and support people who were frequently ignored and shunned by mainstream services or who avoided those services out of fear and suspicion.

Recognising the different knowledges and skills that people brought to the game was important and learning to respect and learn from other professional disciplines improved my clinical skills and the support we could provide together to people often experiencing major life crises. Similarly, working alongside the often hugely talented, creative people with no professional background who worked in the voluntary sector and turned up day after day, often doing the unglamorous work, but engaging and developing relationships in a way that many of us watched with envy. But interprofessional and multiagency working brings its own challenges with regard to different policies and procedures, competing ideas around risk, different underpinning philosophical bases, and professional training and socialisation that can breed distrust and even hostility towards other disciplines.

Thus, I was pleased to see that this book includes chapters on a range of disciplines and addresses many of the issues around interprofessional working and learning. Opening ourselves to the approaches adopted by others, asking questions about how and especially why we do certain things, and grasping opportunities to work alongside and learn from one another can expand our capabilities and help us develop 'team knowledge', ensuring specific expertise is not held in the mind or hands of one individual, who may one day leave!

Finally, as someone involved in policy-related research and aware of how national policies and agendas can shape and sometimes misshape the work being undertaken in the field, I was hoping to find a consideration of relevant policies and guidelines and there is plenty of that in this book, with careful and critical consideration of the key texts.

Working with people in crisis is challenging and immensely important work. It can save people's lives and it can ensure people remain engaged with us to find another, better way forward. There is plenty in this book to get your teeth into and help us think about how we work with people in mental health crises and how we might best make a difference.

Alan Simpson
Professor of Mental Health Nursing
Health Service and Population Research,
Institute of Psychiatry, Psychology and Neuroscience
King's College London
Florence Nightingale Faculty of Nursing, Midwifery and Palliative Care
King's College London
Co-Director, Mental Health Policy Research Unit
Deputy Director, Qualitative Applied Health Research Centre

Abbreviations

AACE	Association of Ambulance Chief Executives		ENP	emergency nurse practitioner
AMHP	Approved Mental Health Professional		ESCMH	essential shared capabilities for mental health
APP	Authorised Professional Practice		EUPD	emotionally unstable personality disorder
ASC	Avon and Somerset Constabulary		HEE	Health Education England
ASW	Approved Social Worker		HMICFR	Her Majesty's Inspectorate of Constabulary and Fire and Rescue Services
BASW	British Association of Social Workers			
BIA	Best Interest Assessor			
BME	Black and minority ethnic		HMIP	Her Majesty's Inspectorate Probation
BSMHFT	Birmingham and Solihull Mental Health Trust		IDVA	Independent Domestic Violence Advisor
CIT	Crisis Intervention Team		IOPC	Independent Office for Police Complaints
CJS	criminal justice system			
CMHT	community mental health teams		IPAP	Intent, Plan, Action and Protective measures
CoP	Code of Practice		IPE	Interprofessional Education
CPD	continuous professional development			
CQC	Care Quality Commission		IPO	Interprofessional Organisation
CRHTT	Crisis Resolution and Home Treatment Team		IPP	Interprofessional Practice
CRPD	Convention on the Rights of Persons with Disabilities		JRCALC	Joint Royal Colleges Ambulance Liaison Committee
			L and D	Liaison and Diversion
CTO	Community Treatment Order		MAPPA	Multi-Agency Public Protection Arrangements
DH	Department of Health		MARAC	Multi-Agency Risk Assessment Conference
DSH	deliberate self-harm			
ECG	electrocardiogram		MCA	Mental Capacity Act
ECHR	European Convention of Human Rights		MDT	multi-disciplinary team
			MHA	Mental Health Act
ED	emergency department		MHFA	Mental Health First Aid
EDT	Emergency Duty Team		MHN	mental health nurse

MHSW	mental health social worker	PICU	psychiatric intensive care unit
MHTA	mental health tactical advisor	PIPS	Peer Inter-Professional Supervision
MSE	Mental State Examination	PLAN	Psychiatric Liaison Accreditation Network
NCALT	National Centre for Applied Learning Technologies	PMVA	Prevention and Management of Violence and Aggression training
NICE	National Institute for Clinical Excellence	PTSD	post-traumatic stress disorder
NMS	neuroleptic malignant syndrome	RCP	Royal College of Psychiatrists
PCDA	Police Constable Degree Apprenticeship	RMO	Responsible Medical Officer
PCE	Police and Criminal Evidence Act 1984	SCW	Social Care Wales
		SWE	Social Work England
PCSO	Police Community Support Officer	TVP	Thames Valley Police
		UWE	University of the West of England
PEQF	Policing Education Qualifications Framework		

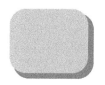

Introduction

Kris Deering and Jo Williams

The Introduction presents the aim of the book, outlining key concepts and policies explored further in each chapter. Interprofessionalism will be introduced alongside the importance of working collaboratively with service users and significant others. An overview of each chapter will be provided to summarise the relevancies of the helping professional. While numerous other professionals could be discussed, those selected reflect the service that may assist within the first crucial 24 hours of a crisis. However, additional professionals will be referred to throughout the book, for when it comes to improving mental health, it is the concern of everyone, despite their profession.

Background

'Collaboration', 'partnership', and 'participation' are terms that have come to embody the modern-day helping professional. Focus is increasingly on enriching patient involvement, including significant others, with service partnerships to support people experiencing mental distress. While collaborative working is recommended for most care settings, the ways service users can be assisted suggest it is most apparent, and possibly needed, in crisis with mental ill-health. Frequently, service users come to the attention of mental health services through different service providers, notably ambulance and police, on account of the urgency surrounding their mental distress (HM Government and Mind, 2014). This means communication and working together across fractured service provision are required to ensure consistent and therapeutic care (Klevan *et al.*, 2018).

When considering a crisis, different connotations can come to mind, based on elevated symptoms, impact on orientation, and risk severities associated with degrees of aggression or violence, self-harm and suicide. These factors, despite somewhat prevalent within crisis do not go to the heart of service user concerns, in that mental health crises involve among things, social events, impairing the quality of life (Agar-Jacomb and Read, 2009; Giménez-Díez *et al.*, 2020). The literature also suggests navigating service provision can by itself compound a crisis, involving disputes highlighting a monetising of concerns about suitable service providers, alongside staff perhaps feeling unprepared and uncertain as to who is best to help (Winters, Magalhaes and Kinsella, 2015).

While a crisis might be understood as an individual and often non-linear journey, the literature proposes that the recovery should include achieving hopefulness, a sense of optimism, a patient voice through joint decision making, reclaiming the past, or connecting with new identities and empowerment (Slade, 2009). Recovery can be more than reducing symptoms and, even with mental illness, involves developing a life that is meaningful. However, critiques observe little data exists about the processes used to reach these outcomes, which sometimes are the antithesis of good crisis scenarios, such as equivocation, sense of invalidation, social concerns surrounding finances, alongside the break-up of intimate relationships, and comorbidity with alcohol and illicit substance use, to name but a few (Biringer *et al.*, 2016; Gillard, Turner and Neffgen, 2015; Paton *et al.*, 2016).

Crisis care can be short-term, embracing momentary support significant to drawing on interpersonal relations with the service user, alongside building bonds with family, friends, and carers (Newransky *et al.*, 2019). These can link to recovery with a respect for autonomous individuals, able to exercise agency with the right to make choices about their lives, although in a crisis this is contingent on the capacity to use personal agency (Swanson *et al.*, 2008). Nonetheless, at times of worthlessness, often seen in crisis scenarios, generating an awareness of involvement in order to acknowledge the person is of value can be beneficial. That is, abandoning hope may signify a crisis, hence shaping connectivity that offsets a sense of being burdensome to others and a purposelessness in life is key to commencing crisis care (Joiner *et al.*, 2012).

Given the importance of collaboration to enable involvement whereby active listening, a non-judgemental stance, and asking for views among other things aids connectivity, the literature suggests such principles equally are significant to collaborate across service providers (Ringdal *et al.*, 2017; King's Fund, 2018). To that end, interprofessionalism involves two or more helping professionals, i.e. a mental health nurse and social worker, ranging from low-level, joint decision making with limited shared resources to multifaceted, fully integrated services, for the purpose of helping an individual (O'Carroll, McSwiggan and Campbell, 2019; Winters, Magalhaes and Kinsella, 2015). Collaboration in terms of interprofessionalism can be defined as:

> involving providers from different specialties, disciplines, or sectors working together to offer complementary services and mutual support, to ensure that individuals receive the most appropriate service from the most appropriate provider in the most suitable location, as quickly as necessary, and with minimal obstacles.
>
> (Craven and Bland, 2006, p. 9)

Despite a wealth of literature about the benefits of interprofessional collaboration, concern remains as to how it might be navigated (HM Government and Mind, 2014). Fragmented pathways to care continue to exist, appearing almost insurmountable when experiencing distress. What is recognised is that, owing to patient disorientation, difficulties arise in how mental distress is disclosed, limiting service navigation. However, mental healthcare persists as being seen somewhat in terms of specialism, in which fractures across services may emulate the dichotomies between law enforcement and patient autonomy, or physical against mental healthcare (Cummins, 2018; Memon *et al.*, 2016).

Government drives, markedly 'parity of esteem', denoting a symmetry of two opposing political forces, attempts to fill a void of disconnected service provision by an equal approach to all healthcare (HM Government, 2011). Yet there manifests a fallacy of relevance, in that physical and mental healthcare, for example, can differ (Mitchell, Hardy and Shiers, 2017). Expertise includes the voices of service users and significant others, something less practical perhaps with other helping disciplines (Soares and Pinto da Costa, 2019). Moreover, care moves beyond mitigating illness as identified with recovery, exploring approaches involving occupation to make life meaningful (Slade, 2009). These features amid others give the impression of unfamiliar care practices raising possible anxieties. This is especially when risks such as suicide are apparent, whereby uncertainty about approaching the topic raises fears that the risk could escalate (Dazzi *et al.*, 2014; RCP, 2020a). Fear of blame also circulates around these concerns, in that errors, sometimes unforeseeable, not only impact on professional reputation, but also bring about managerial scrutiny (Muir-Cochrane, O'Kane and Oster, 2018). Understandably, some professionals struggle with the complex landscape of care, placing the onus on mental health services due to a feeling of being unqualified to assist (Department of Health and Social Care, 2018).

While some services have designated roles with mental healthcare, what this book proposes is that when it comes to improving such health, it is everyone's concern. Mental health acts like a fabric interweaving well-being and society together, thus associated difficulties will be encountered by a range of helping professionals to varying degrees. This text therefore is for those professionals involved in crisis management to help them understand their roles, but also to demystify the roles of other professionals who might be encountered within crisis care. Underpinning each chapter is a position of cultivating partnership and collaboration, commencing with those of the utmost importance: the people experiencing mental distress in need of help. Hence, ways to generate partnership with patients will be explored, involving helping professionals who may be met by the service user. Each chapter will also sketch how the helping professional may aid mental healthcare, gravitating towards partnership with other services with the view that care is cohesive. Also further reading to develop knowledge about the topics highlighted in each chapter is proposed.

Challenges will also be discussed, acknowledging that notwithstanding illustrations of good practice, these are sometimes troublesome, especially when collaboration between services is required (De Sutter *et al.*, 2019). Such challenges will be explored in the context of the professional role, while the concluding chapter will examine ways forward from interpersonal collaboration with service users, and significant others, to services cooperating through approaches enriching whole systems working. What follows is an overview of the Crisis Care Concordat, a prominent policy underpinning the text, and supporting the significance of each chapter. This is to provide an outline about why the helping professionals were selected, their relationships with each other, alongside their professional roles, when supporting a person experiencing a mental health-related crisis.

The Crisis Care Concordat

In response to the variable quality and accessibility of care for people in crisis, despite the best efforts of staff, patients, and significant others to navigate provision, the Mental Health Crisis Care Concordat was developed (HM Government and Mind, 2014). The policy advocates collaboration across providers, hence this is a focal point of the book, in that it supports improving access to services necessary to operationalise crisis management. The policy also recommends improving care and seeking ways to prevent future crises by ensuring people are referred to the appropriate community services. The policy was initiated as it had been long recognised that improvements are needed in how health services, social services and police forces work together (HM Government and Mind, 2014). Problems arise when these services intersect, raising critique of how various helping professionals, despite having supportive roles, interact, alongside concerns about how responsibilities towards the individual are transferred between services (Winters, Magalhaes and Kinsella, 2015). In part, such restrictions manifest owing to different professional practices, perception of job role, and lack of service integration (De Sutter *et al.*, 2019). Hence the Crisis Care Concordat aims that 'NHS [National Health Service] services will also work alongside other system partners including Local Authorities, Police and Ambulance services to deliver comprehensive and accessible local crisis care pathways' (NHS England, 2015).

Crisis care has also been identified in several other UK government policies, notably the Five-Year Forward View for Mental Health (Mental Health Taskforce, 2016), which, among other things, aims to reduce admissions to psychiatric hospitals. Accordingly, to aid delivery of comprehensive and accessible care that limits admissions, the Crisis Care Concordat proposes four principal areas to improve mental healthcare pathways:

- *Access to support before the crisis point* – making sure people with mental health problems can get help 24 hours a day and that when they ask for help, they are taken seriously.
- *Urgent and emergency access to crisis care* – making sure that a mental health crisis is treated with the same urgency as a physical health emergency.
- *Quality of treatment and care when in crisis* – making sure that people are treated with dignity and respect, in a therapeutic environment.
- *Recovery and staying well* – preventing future crises by making sure people are referred to appropriate services.

(HM Government and Mind, 2014)

However, the landscape of care has rapidly altered since the implementation of the Crisis Care Concordat. The impact of the Covid pandemic, for example, has led to more psychiatric hospital admissions and acuity of mental illness (Carr *et al.*, 2021; NHS England, 2020; RCP, 2020c). Though data continues to be gathered, crises have been exacerbated on account of the difficulties with accessing provision (CQC, 2020). Concerns are also raised about service abilities to help with crisis care, alongside prioritising resources based on risk, away from preventative treatment (RCP, 2020a; 2020b). The latter to an extent explains increased hospital admissions, given the increasing demand to contain risks like suicide (Abbas *et al.*, 2020). Moreover, reduction in psychiatric hospital beds and inconsistencies in how services tolerate risks, have resulted in variable provision, difficult to access and navigate, meaning urgent needs are not always met (Davidson, Brophy and Campbell, 2016). Hence, in the spirit of collaboration, another focal point of the text will be unravelling involvement with service users, carers, family and friends. It might not always be possible to achieve the outcomes officially requested in guidelines and policies. Nevertheless, care will be examined in the context of collaboration, with the view that such approaches can help lessen the distress of a crisis, even if it is just for momentary periods.

Before delving into the relevancy of the chapters, it is important to note how services in the text were identified. A recent literature review, conducted by Odejimi, Bagchi and Tadros (2020) on typologies of crisis services in the UK, identifies which service providers to use. However, other services could be discussed, indeed primary care might be fitting, yet as proposed by the review, such services tend not to be employed within the crucial first 24 hours of a crisis especially if the need for help occurs outside of working hours. Also noteworthy is that the arrangement of chapters does not signify a linearity of service provision. That is, a crisis care pathway does not always commence at emergency departments, the first service discussed. As will be shown, multiple pathways exist, stressing the importance of collaboration across services that may support a person in crisis. Finally, each chapter addresses service users and significant others employing terminologies surrounding sex, such as 'he/she' or gender-neutral terms to reflect the diversity of gender. This is to be inclusive of the changing landscape in how people identify themselves, but also in recognition that biological sex can be employed in law and services that aid people experiencing a mental health crisis.

Overview of the book

Chapter 1 Laying the foundations of crisis, interprofessionalism and recovery

How a crisis can be characterised is crucial to understanding the needs of service users, and significant others, but also to realise that when it comes to a crisis and risks, there are likely to be different service interpretations. Hence the focus of this chapter is unpicking collaboration, starting at the micro-level of engaging patients when considering principles of personal recovery, notably via the service user voice, but also discussing conflicts and synthesis with clinical recovery regarding the expertise of the helping professional (Slade, 2009). When exploring collaboration at the macro-level, the chapter will examine current practices surrounding partnership working. Conceptual differences and similarities between services will also be reflected upon that may complement or impede collaboration to meet the standards of the Crisis Care Concordat. Overall, the chapter will present the conceptual foundations to discuss mental health crisis and collaboration in the other chapters to follow, while proposing arguments that will be tackled throughout the book, with suggestions to promote partnership working in Chapter 7.

Chapter 2 Mental health crises in an emergency department

While mental health services could have been an appropriate place to start, considering the topic of the text, access and referrals to mental healthcare occur frequently through an emergency department (ED) within general hospitals. Despite the literature proposing difficulties, such as lack of understanding of mental health needs and perpetuating stigma about self-harm, great opportunities exist in these settings to begin lessening the impact of a crisis (Clarke et al., 2014). Against the backdrop of collaboration, the chapter will explore initiating care to understand the difficulties the service user might be experiencing, hence providing a further reason to start with the ED, given the groundwork, such as assessments, that can occur to commence crisis care. However, crisis management within EDs is complex and fraught with conflicting demands, so the chapter will provide guidance in how care might be promoted while taking account of physical treatment needs, risks, medico-legal frameworks, and other competing pressures. Also touched upon is how ED clinicians can seek assistance from mental health liaison teams based in most large general hospitals, as well as ways to engage with other service providers in order to promote cohesive care.

Chapter 3 The role of mental health services with crisis management

The chapter discusses the role of Crisis Resolution and Home Treatment Teams (CRHTTs), seen sometimes as the last bastion of crisis management before psychiatric hospital admission. When warranted, an important caveat, in that exploration will touch upon a greater tolerance towards risk and crisis severity than perhaps other services, the crisis of a patient is ideally stabilised (Lombardo et al., 2019). Discussion will explore in more depth the topics of Chapter 2, about enriching collaborative care, including with significant others. This will involve, despite being underreported in the UK literature, the value of the Seven-Stage Crisis Intervention Model, as a means of working towards crisis resolution (Roberts and Ottens, 2005).

Medication management and lessening risks associated with mental distress will also be discussed. However, in keeping with the theme of the book, this will be through the lens of participation, noting the importance of patient voice in deciding which risks and care needs are relevant, notwithstanding organisational restraints, while also being an opportunity for personal growth and renewal. That is not to underplay the distress of the crisis, rather through approaches that touch on recovery-based principles, the chapter will illuminate care that is inclusive of personal needs with pharmacological approaches. This is alongside accommodating the liminal state of the crisis consisting of uncertainty about which direction patients take next to reclaim their lives (Boland, 2013). In addition, because CRHTTs tend to be at the forefront of crisis care, complexities will also be discussed surrounding referrals, and in consonance with collaboration, how CRHTTs can assist and guide other services to support an individual in distress.

Chapter 4 Policing the mental health crisis

The police, alongside paramedics, tend to be the first helping professionals on the scene. These services can be called upon, when worried about another or in great despair, seen in terms of a blue light service suggesting rapid responses, when possible, will follow (Mind and Victim Support, 2013). The role of the police is also to review for Section 136 detentions, owing to a person presenting in a public space with characteristics of a mental disorder, requiring a possible place of safety to receive assessment (Wondemaghen, 2021). However, concern exists about police responsibilities as Her Majesty's Inspectorate of Constabulary and Fire and Rescue Services (HMICFR, 2018, p. 3) propose: 'The fact that almost every police force now has its own mental health triage team indicates that there isn't nearly enough emphasis on early intervention and primary care to prevent the need for a crisis response.' This raises questions of whether an absolute linearity of a crisis exists, for it can emerge unexpectedly, meaning no linear journey to work back from, to prevent the crisis materialising in the first place. Notable issues surrounding loss of employment, friendships, and intimate relationships are relative to the individual specific to a point in time and place, hence may accumulate into a crisis unpredictably (White *et al.*, 2019). That does not downplay the need for prevention but owing to the fledgling landscape of mental health preventative measures, police will have some form of involvement with crises in the foreseeable future (Watson and Fulambarker, 2012).

Nevertheless, like other services, it is recognised that constabularies are stretched with competing demands, causing conflicts in which the goal of upholding law and order can be diluted to accommodate unfamiliar roles (Compton *et al.*, 2014). These aspects will be discussed, including the expectation of the service and, despite competing demands, evidence of good practice to aid people in a crisis does exist (Mental Health Network, 2015). Granted, this will include street triage but also ways police officers can collaborate with an individual alongside carers, friends, and families to lessen the upset and impact of the crisis. Onus on the officer is less about identifying mental health conditions but attributes such as compassion and care can still be provided as some evidence will show. In addition, there will be discussion of working in partnership with other services, as through such partnerships the burden on the force can lessen, decreasing the feeling of being isolated with the sense they are primarily responsible for a person in crisis (Murray *et al.*, 2021).

Chapter 5 The role of the paramedic in mental health crisis care

Paramedics, like the police, can be called upon first, owing to the urgency believed to exist with the mental health crisis. Accordingly, paramedics and the police are sometimes seen as the adhesive between more fixed statutory mental health services, without which, awareness of a crisis might not come to their attention. Traditionally, the scope of paramedics' practice has been pre-hospital emergency care, however, it is now recognised that paramedics address gaps within health provision, in which crisis care is one such gap. As a result, the role of the paramedic has broadened to be more inclusive of mental healthcare (Emond, O'Meara and Bish, 2019), while the London Ambulance Service (2020) callouts for suicide-related incidents increased to an average of 37 per day compared to 22 in 2019.

Time constraints and lack of treatment options have led to the suggestion that the paramedic role is to transport patients in crisis to the most appropriate care setting (Moskovitz, Sapadin and Guttenberg, 2020). However, the chapter will suggest that the capabilities of paramedics go beyond transportation, involving opportunities to initiate crisis care through collaborative means (Moskovitz, Sapadin and Guttenberg, 2020). Paramedics have increasingly important roles with the assessment and early management of self-harm, displaying great abilities of understanding and coordinating with other agencies (Cook, 2019; NICE, 2004). Despite these key attributes, as a first responder, paramedics also experience significant exposure to mental distress (Kus, Henderson and Batt, 2019). Given such exposure, the literature proposes the need for partnership working, to ensure responsibilities are shared and to lessen the burden of stress (Regehr *et al.*, 2002). These issues among others will be discussed. In addition, despite perhaps a lack of physical needs at the time, crisis situations can be seen by patients and significant others as emergencies, requiring empathetic ways to address concerns. But also, depending on the level of urgency, signposting can be a helpful intervention, to raise awareness of more suitable service providers (Irving *et al.*, 2016).

Chapter 6 The role of mental health social workers in crisis work: values, responsibilities, powers and duties

Social services play a key role in managing risk and complexity in participation with people experiencing overwhelming health and social difficulties. Social workers make up several multidisciplinary mental health teams, and traditionally, this could be as an Approved Social Worker (ASW) in England and Wales (Stone, 2019). The purpose of the role was to have deciding authority in who was detainable under the Mental Health Act (1983). Following the 2007 revision of the Act, scope broadened to include other professionals under the role of Approved Mental Health Professional (AMHP) (Mental Health Act, 2007). However, the role continues to be one somewhat embraced by the social worker profession (BASW, 2016). As a result, the chapter builds on legal frameworks previously discussed, contemplated when a person is in crisis. This will include least restrictive practices, risks, outlining the definition of mental disorder and responsibilities with safeguarding and mental capacity. Because the endpoint of assessment can be exploring the place for legislation to preserve patient safety, AMHPs have an integral role to advise on harnessing least restrictive practices, particularly to lessen hospital admissions. Nevertheless, conflicts can occur involving opposing views about safety and patient needs (Simpson, 2020). Hence ways to cope with such conflicts will be explored alongside collaboration with patients and significant others, including other service providers, when supporting a person in distress.

Chapter 7 Collaboration and whole system working

Despite the rapidly changing landscape of mental healthcare, the Crisis Care Concordat is a vision that sets the standard for partnership working. Drawing on previous discussions, the chapter will examine ways to work towards this goal, progressing from interpersonal collaboration to tying provision together to promote whole systems working. While different professional roles exist, conceivably there is a shared ethic of helping another in distress, and importance will be placed on this notion that despite differences, all helping professionals have a similar aim to help another.

Touching on the Department of Health's (2004) ten essential shared capabilities, a framework for the whole of the mental health workforce, the chapter will outline innovations, notably through the values of building social relationships between service providers, whereby collaboration is not out of necessity of a crisis but to lessen future conflicts. As a result, such collaboration ensures the focus, whenever possible, remains on patient care. Given the fractures in provision, particularly surrounding commissioning, also explored will be the fact that some barriers might require structural reform at a national level (Moreno et al., 2020). However, to inform such change requires evidence of innovations that promote patient care, suggesting sometimes a need to circumnavigate organisational boundaries to build partnerships. That is, while limitations are recognised, it will be proposed these should not hinder grassroots partnership building that may lessen the patient's suffering by navigating service provision (Smith et al., 2017).

An outline of the text is provided, touching on collaboration with patients and significant others, but also service providers, on the variable crisis pathways in operation. Each provider's role is summarised to show the significance of their role, recognising that despite other provisions, these tend to be involved within the first crucial 24 hours of a crisis. The Crisis Care Concordat with partnership working is highlighted, given that mental health and society are bound together, suggesting professionals illustrated in the policy and text will encounter associated difficulties to varying degrees. Hence partnerships are required to share responsibilities and lessen the burden of stress. It is also proposed that all professionals hold a moral standing to help a person in distress, providing the basis to overcome organisational restraints and feasibly work more collaboratively together. These aspects among others will be further explored throughout the text, commencing with theories and ideas about crisis, collaboration, and recovery in Chapter 1.

Further reading

- **Crisis Care Concordat:**
  https://www.crisiscareconcordat.org.uk/
- **Five-Year Forward View:**
  https://www.england.nhs.uk/wp-content/uploads/2016/02/Mental-Health-Taskforce-FYFV-final.pdf
- **King's Fund, *Joined Up Listening*:**
  https://www.kingsfund.org.uk/publications/joined-up-listening-integrated-care-and-patient-insight
- **Mental Health Network, Briefing Paper:**
  https://www.nhsconfed.org/~/media/Confederation/Files/Publications/Documents/mental-health-crisis-care.pdf
- **Mind Mental Health Charity, Crises Reports:**
  https://www.mind.org.uk/about-us/our-policy-work/reports-and-guides/crisis-care-reports/
- **NHS England, Integrated Care Recommendations:**
  https://www.england.nhs.uk/integratedcare/

References

Abbas, M.J., Kronenberg, G., McBride, M., Chari, D., Alam, F., Mukaetova-Ladinska, E., Al-Uzri, M. and Brugha, T. (2020) The early impact of the Covid-19 pandemic on acute care mental health services. *Psychiatric Services.* Available at: https://ps.psychiatryonline.org/doi/10.1176/appi.ps.202000467?url_ver=Z39.88-2003andrfr_id=ori:rid:crossref.organdrfr_dat=cr_pub%20%200pubmed (accessed 10 February 2021).

Agar-Jacomb, K. and Read, J. (2009) Mental health crisis services: What do service users need when in crisis? *Journal of Mental Health*, 18(2), 99–110.

BASW (British Association of Social Workers) (2016) *The Role of the Social Worker in Adult Mental Health Services.* Available at: https://www.basw.co.uk/system/files/resources/basw_112306-10_0.pdf (accessed 10 January 2021).

Biringer, E., Davidson, L., Sundfòr, B., Ruud, T. and Borg, M. (2016) Experiences of support in working toward personal recovery goals: A collaborative, qualitative study. *BMC Psychiatry*, 16(1), 426.

Boland, T. (2013) Towards an anthropology of critique: The modern experience of liminality and crisis. *Anthropological Theory*, 13(3), 222–239.

Carr, M.J., Steeg, S., Webb, R.T., Kapur, N., Chew-Graham, C.A., Abel, K.M., Hope, H., Pierce, M. and Ashcroft, D.M. (2021) Effects of the COVID-19 pandemic on primary care-recorded mental illness and self-harm episodes in the UK: A population-based cohort study. *The Lancet: Public Health*, 6(2), 124–135.

Clarke, D., Usick, R., Sanderson, A., Giles-Smith, L. and Baker, J. (2014) Emergency department staff attitudes towards mental health consumers: A literature review and thematic content analysis. *International Journal of Mental Health Nursing*, 23(3), 273–284.

Compton, M.T., Bakeman, R., Broussard, B., Hankerson-Dyson, D., Husbands, L., Krishan, S., Stewart-Hutto, T., D'Orio, B.M., … and Watson, A.C. (2014) The police-based Crisis Intervention Team (CIT) model: I. Effects on officers' knowledge, attitudes, and skills. *Psychiatric Services*, 65(4), 517–522.

Cook, A. (2019) Taking a holistic approach to acute mental health crisis. *Journal of Paramedic Practice: The Clinical Monthly or Emergency Care Professional*, 11(10), 426–432.

CQC (Care Quality Commission) (2020) Community Mental Health Survey: Statistical Release. Available at: https://www.cqc.org.uk/sites/default/files/20201124_cmh20_statisticalrelease.pdf (accessed 3 January 2021).

Craven, M.A. and Bland, R. (2006) Better practices in collaborative mental health care: An analysis of the evidence base. *Canadian Journal of Psychiatry*, 51(6), 1–74.

Cummins, I. (2018) The impact of austerity on mental health service provision: A UK perspective. *International Journal of Environmental Research and Public Health*, 15(6), 1145–1156.

Davidson, G., Brophy, L. and Campbell, J. (2016) Risk, recovery and capacity: Competing or complementary approaches to mental health social work. *Australian Social Work*, 69(2), 158–168.

Dazzi, T., Gribble, R., Wessely, S. and Fear, N.T. (2014) Does asking about suicide and related behaviours induce suicidal ideation? What is the evidence? *Psychological Medicine*, 44(16), 3361–3363.

Department of Health (2004) *The Ten Essential Shared Capabilities: A Framework for the Whole of the Mental Health Workforce*. London: Department of Health.

Department of Health and Social Care (2018) *Modernising the Mental Health Act: Final Report from the Independent Review*. Available at: https://www.gov.uk/government/publications/modernising-the-mental-health-act-final-report-from-the-independent-review (accessed 11 December 2020).

De Sutter, M., De Sutter, A., Sundahl, N., Declercq, T. and Decat, P. (2019) Interprofessional collaboration reduces the burden of caring for patients with mental illnesses in primary healthcare: A realist evaluation study. *The European Journal of General Practice*, 25(4), 236–242.

Emond, K., O'Meara, P. and Bish, M. (2019) Paramedic management of mental health related presentations: A scoping review. *Journal of Mental Health*, 28(1), 89–96.

Gillard, S., Turner, K. and Neffgen, M. (2015) Understanding recovery in the context of lived experience of personality disorders: A collaborative, qualitative research study. *BMC Psychiatry*, 15(1), 183.

Giménez-Díez, D., Maldonado Alía, R., Rodríguez Jiménez, S., Granel, N., Torrent Solà, L. and Bernabeu-Tamayo, M.D. (2020) Treating mental health crises at home: Patient satisfaction with home nursing care. *Journal of Psychiatric and Mental Health Nursing*, 27(3), 246–257.

HM Government (2011) No health without mental health. Available at: https://assets.publishing.service.gov.uk/government/uploads/system/uploads/attachment_data/file/138253/dh_124058.pdf (accessed 10 June 2021).

HM Government and Mind (2014) *The Crisis Care Concordat.* Available at: https://www.crisiscareconcordat.org.uk/ (accessed 10 December 2020).

HMICFR (Her Majesty's Inspectorate of Constabulary and Fire and Rescue Services) (2018) Policing and mental health: Picking up the pieces. Available at: https://www.justiceinspectorates.gov.uk/hmicfrs/wp-content/uploads/policing-and-mental-health-picking-up-the-pieces.pdf (accessed 5 January 2020).

Irving, A., O'Hara, R., Johnson, M., Harris, A. and Baker, K. (2016) Pilot evaluation of utilising mental health nurses in the management of ambulance service patients with mental health problems. *Emergency Medicine Journal,* 33(9), 677.

Joiner, T.E., Ribeiro, J.D. and Silva, C. (2012) Nonsuicidal self-injury, suicidal behavior, and their co-occurrence as viewed through the lens of the interpersonal theory of suicide. *Current Directions in Psychological Science: A Journal of the American Psychological Society,* 21(5), 342–347.

King's Fund (2018) *Joined-up Listening: Integrated Care and Patient Insight.* Available at: https://www.kingsfund.org.uk/publications/joined-up-listening-integrated-care-and-patient-insight (accessed 12 December 2020).

Klevan, T., Karlsson, B., Ness, O., Grant, A. and Ruud, T. (2018) Between a rock and a softer place: A discourse analysis of helping cultures in crisis resolution teams. *Qualitative Social Work: Research and Practice,* 17(2), 252–267.

Kus, L., Henderson, L. and Batt, A.M. (2019) Empathy in paramedic practice: An overview. *Journal of Paramedic Practice: The Clinical Monthly for Emergency Care Professionals,* 11(4), 1–5.

Lombardo, C., Santos, M., Van Bortel, T., Croos, R., Arensman, E. and Kar Ray, M. (2019) Decision-making in crisis resolution and home treatment teams: The AWARE framework. *BJPsych Bulletin,* 43(2), 61–66.

London Ambulance Service (2020) Status. 28 October. Available at: https://twitter.com/Ldn_Ambulance/status/1321566876732952581 (accessed 13 May 2021).

Memon, A., Taylor, K., Mohebati, L.M., Sundin, J., Cooper, M., Scanlon, T. and de Visser, R. (2016) Perceived barriers to accessing mental health services among black and minority ethnic (BME) communities: A qualitative study in Southeast England. *BMJ Open,* 6(11), 1–9.

Mental Health Act (1983) Available at: https://www.legislation.gov.uk/ukpga/1983/20/contents (accessed 8 January 2021).

Mental Health Act (2007) Available at: https://www.legislation.gov.uk/ukpga/2007/12/contents (accessed 8 January 2021).

Mental Health Network (2015) Mental health and policing: Improving crisis care. Available at: https://www.nhsconfed.org/-/media/Confederation/Files/public-access/Briefing-279-Mental-health-and-policing-final-26-Jan.pdf (accessed 8 January 2021).

Mental Health Taskforce (2016) Five-Year Forward View for Mental Health. Available at: https://www.england.nhs.uk/wp-content/uploads/2016/02/Mental-Health-Taskforce-FYFV-final.pdf (accessed 12 June 2021).

Mind and Victim Support (2013) Police and mental health. Available at: https://www.mind.org.uk/media-a/4356/2013-12-03-mind_police_final_web.pdf (accessed 3 December 2020).

Mitchell, A.J., Hardy, S. and Shiers, D. (2017) Parity of esteem: Addressing the inequalities between mental and physical healthcare. *BJPsych Advances,* 23(3), 196–205.

Moreno, C., Wykes, T., Galderisi, S., Nordentoft, M., Crossley, N., Jones, N., Cannon, M., Correll, C.U., Byrne, L., ... and Arango, C. (2020) How mental health care should change as a consequence of the COVID-19 pandemic. *The Lancet: Psychiatry*, 7(9), 813–824.

Moskovitz, J., Sapadin, J. and Guttenberg, M. (2020) Interfacility ambulance transport of mental health patients. *Journal of the American College of Emergency Physicians Open*, 1(3), 173–182.

Muir-Cochrane, E., O'Kane, D. and Oster, C. (2018) Fear and blame in mental health nurses' accounts of restrictive practices: Implications for the elimination of seclusion and restraint. *International Journal of Mental Health Nursing*, 27(5), 1511–1521.

Murray, J., Heyman, I., Dougall, N., Wooff, A., Aston, E. and Enang, I. (2021) Co-creation of five key research priorities across law enforcement and public health: A methodological example and outcomes. *Journal of Psychiatric and Mental Health Nursing*, 28(1), 3–15.

Newransky, C.M., Monti, K. and Lombe, M. (2019) Addressing the treatment gap for individuals with serious mental illness: Can a short-term crisis and transitional intervention impact psychiatric and medical service utilization? *Best Practices in Mental Health*, 15(1), 1–19.

NHS England (2015) *Crisis and Acute Mental Health Services*. Available at: https://www.england.nhs.uk/mental-health/adults/crisis-and-acute-care/ (accessed 17 December 2020).

NHS England (2020) NHS Mental Health Dashboard December 2020, publication Period: Quarter 1 2020/21. Available at: https://www.england.nhs.uk/mental-health/taskforce/imp/mh-dashboard/ (accessed 5 February 2021).

NICE (National Institute for Clinical Excellence) (2004) *Self-harm: The Short Term Physical and Psychological Management and Secondary Prevention of Self-harm in Primary and Secondary Care*. Available at: https://www.nice.org.uk/guidance/CG16 (accessed 10 February 2021).

O'Carroll, V., McSwiggan, L. and Campbell, M. (2019) Practice educators' attitudes and perspectives of interprofessional collaboration and interprofessional practice learning for students: A mixed-methods case study. *Journal of Interprofessional Care*, 33(5), 414–423.

Odejimi, O., Bagchi, D. and Tadros, G. (2020) Typology of psychiatric emergency services in the United Kingdom: A narrative literature review. *BMC Psychiatry*, 20(1), 587.

Paton, F., Wright, K., Ayre, N., Dare, C., Johnson, S., Lloyd-Evans, B., Simpson, A., Webber, M. and Meader, N. (2016) Improving outcomes for people in mental health crisis: A rapid synthesis of the evidence for available models of care. *Health Technology Assessment*, 20(3), 1–162.

Regehr, C., Goldberg, G. and Hughes, J. (2002) Exposure to human tragedy, empathy, and trauma in ambulance paramedics. *American Journal of Orthopsychiatry*, 72(4), 505–513.

Ringdal, M., Chaboyer, W., Ulin, K., Bucknall, T. and Oxelmark, L. (2017) Patient preferences for participation in patient care and safety activities in hospitals. *BMC Nursing*, 16(1), 69–77.

Roberts, A.R. and Ottens, A.J. (2005) The seven-stage crisis intervention model: A road map to goal attainment, problem solving, and crisis resolution. *Brief Treatment and Crisis Intervention*, 5(4), 329–339.

RCP (Royal College of Psychiatrists) (2020a) *Self-harm and Suicide in Adults: Final Report of the Patient Safety Group*. Available at: https://www.rcpsych.ac.uk/docs/

default-source/improving-care/better-mh-policy/college-reports/college-report-cr229-self-harm-and-suicide.pdf?sfvrsn=b6fdf395_10 (accessed 11 January 2021).

RCP (Royal College of Psychiatrists) (2020b) Briefing analysis of second COVID-19 RCPsych member survey – indirect harm. Available at: https://www.rcpsych.ac.uk/docs/default-source/about-us/covid-19/second-rcpsych-covid-member-survey-summary—indirect-harms.pdf?sfvrsn=13a88d7d_4 (accessed 2 February 2021).

RCP (Royal College of Psychiatrists) (2020c) *COVID-19: Guidance for Community and Inpatient Services*. Available at: https://www.rcpsych.ac.uk/about-us/responding-to-covid-19/responding-to-covid-19-guidance-for-clinicians/community-and-inpatient-services (accessed 3 January 2021).

Simpson, M. (2020) A structured narrative literature review of approved mental health professional detention decisions: An infusion of morality. *Practice*, 32(4), 285–300.

Slade, M. (2009) *Personal Recovery and Mental Illness: A Guide for Mental Health Professionals*. Cambridge: Cambridge University Press.

Smith, A., Fressoli, M., Abrol, D., Arond, E. and Ely, A. (2017) *Grassroots Innovation Movements*. London: Routledge.

Soares, R. and Pinto da Costa, M. (2019) Experiences and perceptions of police officers concerning their interactions with people with serious mental disorders for compulsory treatment. *Frontiers in Psychiatry*, 10, 187.

Stone, K. (2019) Approved mental health professionals and detention: An exploration of professional differences and similarities. *Practice*, 31(2), 83–96.

Swanson, J.W., Swartz, M.S., Elbogen, E.B., Van Dorn, R.A., Wagner, H.R., Moser, L.A., Wilder, C. and Gilbert, A.R. (2008) Psychiatric advance directives and reduction of coercive crisis interventions. *Journal of Mental Health*, 17(3), 255–267.

Watson, A.C. and Fulambarker, A.J. (2012) The Crisis Intervention Team model of police response to mental health crises: A primer for mental health practitioners. *Best Practices in Mental Health*, 8(2), 71–81.

White, C., Goldberg, V., Hibdon, J. and Weisburd, D. (2019) Understanding the role of service providers, land use, and resident characteristics on the occurrence of mental health crisis calls to the police. *Journal of Community Psychology*, 47(8), 1961–1982.

Winters, S., Magalhaes, L. and Kinsella, E.A. (2015) Interprofessional collaboration in mental health crisis response systems: Scoping review. *Disability and Rehabilitation*, 37(23), 2212–2224.

Wondemaghen, M. (2021) Policing mental illness: Police use of Section 136. Perspectives from police and mental-health nurses. *Medicine, Science, and the Law*. Early View, 1–9.

1 Laying the foundations of crisis, interprofessionalism and recovery

Stevie Morris, Jo Williams and Kris Deering

Current crisis management practices present professionals with a complex terrain. Therefore, this introductory chapter seeks to explore and enhance the readers' understanding of definitions and terminology commonly employed when working in healthcare together with other providers, to support a person experiencing a mental health crisis. This will include terms 'crisis' and 'recovery' with how services are structured to meet service user needs.

The section relating to recovery perspectives will explore and include the service user experience in relation to personal recovery, in what might be meaningful to the person, but there will also be consideration of the perspectives of service providers, in terms of clinical recovery, which draws on the expertise of the helping professional. Notions of risk and service provision will be discussed, and the challenges presented by fragmented service provision will also be contemplated. Understanding the needs of service user experiences is key to assisting in alleviating a crisis and each experience will be individual and uniquely characterised. Hence the chapter will enable the reader to realise that when an individual is experiencing 'a crisis' and 'presenting with risks', there are likely to be different individual and service interpretations.

Another aim of this chapter is to extend understanding of the wider landscape surrounding collaborative crisis work and interprofessionalism. We seek to unpick what is understood to be collaborative current working practices and how locating equilibrium via co-production, a form of partnership building, helps professionals work together with service users to synthesise their recovery and meet the standards of the Crisis Care Concordat.

The chapter will conclude with an overview and discussion surrounding the spectrum model, which presents the stages of a crisis experience and considers that stages, rather than focusing on definitions, may be a more helpful way to identify how and when services can support a person in crisis. By considering stages, exploration can be facilitated of the differing ways a crisis can be experienced, according to service users and significant others. Overall, the chapter will present conceptual grounds about crisis and collaboration, creating a foundation to underpin the later chapters on service providers and their roles in aiding a person experiencing a mental health crisis.

Introduction

Readers will be drawn to this text from diverse backgrounds and for a range of reasons. You may be a student/professional undergoing training or an experienced practitioner seeking to explore further and extend interprofessional working practices. Maybe you have grappled with your own mental health challenges, supported a family member or friend and are seeking to understand how professionals 'define' a mental health crisis, alongside the rationale for the approaches employed in helping and supporting those 'in crisis'.

What is not in doubt is that the challenging nature of working in crisis management and the current practices present professionals with a complex terrain. Yet this terrain is not solely experienced by professionals; service users and their families find that when experiencing a crisis, navigating the fragmented service provision and different crisis interpretations can cause confusion and exacerbate symptoms of distress, thus impacting on the person in crisis and those around them seeking to assist them.

The experience of crisis in itself is highly personal and therefore unique to an individual and is characterised by an array of feelings and behaviours. The response and actions of those around the person 'in crisis' will determine whether outcomes are perceived positively, fulfil needs and help facilitate recovery or contribute negatively to the individual's experience leading to, and resulting in, detrimental impact.

In acknowledging that readers arrive at this text having experienced unique journeys, this chapter will introduce and explore definitions of crisis and recovery (personal and clinical). In doing so, we recognise that personal and clinical/professional perspectives regarding these concepts differ, yet can be synthesised. Notably, through collaboration, a compromise is sought whenever possible, involving the expertise of service users and professionals to find out what might help.

Defining terms: what is a crisis?

Before seeking to explore the complex nuances of personal and professional perspectives of the aforementioned concepts, a useful starting point is to consider and define commonly used terminology; first, 'crisis' and then 'recovery', in their varying guises. This will enable the reader to gain a grasp of the often complex and frequently used terminology employed by individuals, groups and stakeholders throughout this text and in practice (Paton *et al.*, 2016).

The term 'crisis' generically, without supplementary terms such as 'personal' and/or 'mental health', is considered 'a period of intense difficulty or danger' and 'a time when a difficult or important decision needs to be made' (*Oxford English Dictionary*, 2021). Greene *et al.* (2000) espouse the Chinese translation of the term as consisting of two separate characters: danger and opportunity.

It is a term used interchangeably to describe a plethora of events across local, national and international platforms, including the financial crisis, natural disasters, conflict and war, crises of a humanitarian nature and very recently, the Covid-19 pandemic which has created a health and social crisis of significant magnitude (Sukut and Ayhan Balik, 2021). However, when we use the term in context, for example, a mental health crisis, this contributes to a shift in understanding and can broaden interpretations of the event. It also leads to a different response, in which context helps us to understand an experience and prompts us to consider what the antecedent(s) might be and how the crisis might be defined.

The work of Caplan (1964) suggests that a crisis occurs when a person is confronted with a problem that cannot be (re)solved. These presenting, apparently unresolvable issues, result in escalated feelings of anxiety and tension, a subsequent state of emotional distress and a compromised ability to function, often for significantly extended periods. Understandably, an individual experiencing such events may struggle to employ effective coping mechanisms and perceive their situation as intolerably difficult, exceeding their personal reservoir of resources and familiar coping strategies, to enable resolution (James and Gilliland, 2005; Roberts and Ottens, 2005). In recognising that the experience of a crisis is often distressing for an individual (and for those around them), it may lead to the person presenting as a risk to themselves and/or others. Those who seek to support and work alongside a person who is experiencing a crisis and provide interventions can create opportunities to promote personal strengths, maintaining or generating new coping strategies relevant to the service user (Peterson and Seligman, 2004).

Heath (2006) set out a range of best practices for crisis communication aimed at media and public relations groups and herein considered the aspect of understanding the narrative of those involved with mental health crisis care. The core concept of accepting the narrative of the lived experience of the person connected to the crisis was proposed, but also the requirement to focus on working with others rather than 'controlling' the presenting problem. As later chapters will attest, this echoes with the best practices aspired to by Crisis Resolution Home Treatment Team (CRHTT) practitioners (Morant *et al.*, 2017), yet the reality experienced by those attempting to access support via services highlights inconsistencies throughout their contact with helping professionals (Mind, 2014). The multifaceted definition of crisis creates differing expectations and subsequent non-alignment between patient and professional/services. Hence, it is through this prism that helping professionals must seek to work when supporting a person experiencing, and presenting with, a mental health crisis.

In seeking to understand the dissonance enveloping the term crisis, there are four key stakeholder perspectives to consider: (1) the patient; (2) families and carers; (3) the helping professionals; and (4) the service commissioners/ policy-makers (NICE, 2016) and it is important to understand the impact on practices present today. Over the last decade, mounting evidence points to the disparities and inconsistencies regarding the services available to the public for mental health-related crises (CQC, 2015: 2020; Mind, 2020; Molodynski *et al.*, 2020). Lavoie (2018) purports that service users view CRHTT practitioners as primary stakeholders. Mental health and/or CRHTT practitioners may use the term crisis to describe the necessity for admission to a psychiatric inpatient unit, or the likelihood of a serious untoward incident, including death (Lloyd-Evans and Johnson, 2014).

In contrast, non-mental health professionals may consider the term to mean something more ethereal, such as, no longer seeing a way through an overwhelming difficulty and needing support or guidance to overcome the insurmountable obstacle ahead (NICE, 2011; 2016). This presents a whole spectrum of what a crisis might entail; its duration, precipitating/causal events and the severity of outcome for individuals and others. Will a single definition for crisis in the context of mental health ever suffice or justly represent and empower all key stakeholders? The literature suggests a universally meaningful definition is far from being accepted in practice and therefore the notion of a 'spectrum of mental health crisis' would be more fitting and appropriate to promote open dialogue, in the hope of creating a shared understanding between all the parties concerned, helping to narrow the gaps currently experienced by all involved in crisis care.

Personal and clinical recovery

Taking into consideration the personal experiences of a crisis (highlighted in the spectrum model) links to recovery, a term that has evolved since the 1980s in mental healthcare (Deegan, 1988). Recovery differs from traditional views about the absence of disease and involves cultivating a meaningful life, regardless of mental health difficulties (Anthony, 1993). Mental health is multifaceted, and mental health illness, although debilitating, does not mean that every part of life is affected, nor does it mean that owing to illness, the person has to stop living, especially when living includes exploring what might improve life for the person (Repper and Perkins, 2003). Distressing symptoms of illness are not ignored, but improving the quality of life led by service user views, alongside clinical treatment, is the key to recovery-orientated care. Despite some commonalities like risk, i.e. self-harm, and diagnosis, each patient will have their own unique interpretation of what led to a crisis incident. Hence, alongside significant others, a patient may have a deeper understanding of what may help or at least of the life stressors involved that led to requiring assistance (Deering *et al.*, 2021).

Recovery aligns to a person-centred approach adopted in healthcare, placing the hopes, wishes and needs of the person experiencing mental health difficulties at the forefront of care (Storm and Edwards, 2013). Person-centred approaches empower by drawing on patient agency to consider personal needs, while participation in decision making generates a sense of ownership over care (Pulvirenti, McMillan and Lawn, 2014). Although achieving personal care goals is important, a contradiction might materialise in which the patient is unable to keep themselves and/or others safe, in that the risk of suicide, for example, outweighs upholding patient autonomy. Autonomy surrounds the right to enact personal choices permissible within law, yet extreme distress can limit the abilities to reason the choices available. Focus in such scenarios can deviate from person-centred care to prioritising risk reduction to promote the immediate safety of the person. Hence crisis care can gravitate towards paternalism, in that the professional decides what is best for the patient despite possible disagreements (Ruggeri and Tansella, 2012).

Great distress can impact on autonomy, meaning decision making to the degree to which patients are accustomed can be difficult to achieve. Patients may seek to relinquish some control so that the helping professional can make immediate decisions about care, for the mental distress is clouding their abilities to make choices (Deering *et al.*, 2019), thus placing the onus on the patient to make decisions can, on occasion, inadvertently lead to further distress. Nevertheless, in the spirit of recovery, professionals do not hold control permanently and 'hand back' as soon as possible in a manner tolerable to the patient. Finding a balance is complex, particularly between paternalism and 'responsibilisation'. The latter is where patients and significant others are rendered responsible for care as part of recovery practices, and when resisted, failure is seen on the part of the patient, and their loved ones, not the service provider (Roy and Buchanan, 2016). Given societal views about the ills of institutionalisation involving a helplessness owing to over-reliance on statutory support, autonomy in a way can be the justification as a recovery approach to not provide care (Brown, 2021). By doing so, it is seen to give back autonomy and responsibility, an approach adopted in some NHS trusts to lessen the impact of people who frequently use healthcare services owing to their mental health difficulties (Centre for Mental Health, 2021).

It appears aspects like paternalism and responsibilisation are something difficult when imposed, resulting in patients not having a voice in what will be helpful. Recovery therefore appears to have different faces, set by patients, or professionals, while perhaps significant others are caught in the middle. Yet studies have shown that while different views about treatment exist, a civic consciousness may remain; a responsibility in a social sense that people, for the most part, desire to connect with others (Brown, 2021). It is here we find a middle ground. By being curious, connectivity can occur in which demonstrating a genuine interest in the patient is reciprocated with openness about the crisis situation (Deering *et al.*, 2021). Moreover, recovery is more than the crisis itself and concerns the life beyond the crisis incident, working towards regaining or establishing new ways of coping. Recovery is not something that necessarily occurs in the first crucial 24 hours when in immediate need of help, but all helping professionals can contribute to set the recovery journey in motion through how they interact with the patient (Gregory and Thompson, 2013).

In light of the different faces of recovery, Slade (2009) identified that it can be clinical, as well as personal. Clinical recovery is open to critique, particularly about a medical perspective of illness, involving specific criteria about what is illness, and what is treatment, defined by the expertise of helping professionals (Barber, 2012). But in crisis management, as will be seen in the following chapters, there is division over this view. A number of professionals feel unqualified to assist, citing a lack of expertise and obligation to help, owing to lack of mental health resources. Expertise in these cases implies specialised knowledge, and that alone is key to managing mental health difficulties. But mental healthcare is far more than knowledge of conditions and treatment options, and even for those with such knowledge, difficulties surrounding risk and uncertainty about care options may remain. While some health conditions are resolved with expertise, for example, surgical issues, mental health difficulties go beyond solely medical treatment and as the following will show, this does not downplay the need for helping professionals, for expertise can come in different guises.

In Chapter 7, you will note patients and loved ones identify the ethics of mental healthcare to concern mutual respect, being non-judgemental, and listening with interest (Department of Health, 2004). In terms of clinical recovery, these are attributes that most helping professionals have, and the expertise used in crisis scenarios. Granted, when applied to mental health services, clinical recovery includes reducing symptoms requiring understanding of prescribed medicines and talking therapies that align with patient needs and conditions (O'Keeffe *et al.*, 2018), but in the first 24 hours of addressing a crisis, we propose expertise comes from kindness, demonstrating active listening and interest in understanding the situation. Another attribute is reflexivity, reviewing how interactions with service users can be improved, be it from the helping professional, their team, or overall service provider. All professions in this text engage in different methods of reflective practice, as a process of continuous learning, and as part of professional development to ensure the provision of a quality service (Cook, 2019). Hence, while mental health knowledge is required in specific services, clinical recovery involving therapeutic engagement is something we believe can be adopted in a crisis, whatever the profession involved.

In contrast, personal recovery surrounds expertise by experience, touching on how mental health difficulties are personally experienced, alongside individual beliefs about the way life can be improved (Tse *et al.*, 2019). Expertise by experience brings in the view that, in addition to theoretical or scientific knowledge – associated with clinical recovery – there is a knowledge based on experience, which enriches and brings new perspectives to professional expertise. Personal recovery includes the views of the patient and significant others about the causes of the crisis, and moves beyond a medicalised focus, notably a relapse in illness. Instead, personal recovery considers, like the stress vulnerability model in Chapter 3, that there are personal life events and difficulties leading to the crisis (Ruggeri and Tansella, 2012). Many readers of this text will have experiences of heartbreak, bereavement and difficulties at work, and when recalling them, it could be that these events had a significant impact on their mental health. It is likely then, that equally such reasons may be precipitating factors that lead to patients experiencing crisis.

When helping professionals attempt to understand the world of the patient and their points of view, opportunities arise, leading to personal growth and development (Tse *et al.*, 2016). Feedback that the patient's views matter can inspire hope, and, for momentary periods in a crisis situation, can provide a space to consider other options. This is important when the person is speaking of wanting to end their life. It can seem such opportunities are rare, particularly with immediate safety concerns. However, small opportunities can still be sought to provide the patient with a voice and make decisions that are tolerable for them and limit harm. In terms of personal and clinical recovery, rather than distinction, the approaches can be interchangeable practices, employed relative to the crisis severity specific to a point in time, and contingent on the needs of the patient (Slade *et al.*, 2014).

What might constitute a crisis?

The question of what constitutes a crisis very much depends on the lens a person is viewing it through, and positionality is key. From a professional perspective, positionality refers to the stance or positioning of the person relative to their professional and social context in relation to others, including a person, a community, an organisation, or group. The position adopted by the professional will impact on the experience of the person seeking help, yet professionals do not usually act in isolation and the role and functioning of their employing organisation will contribute to their response. As you explore the following chapters, what will become apparent is that the provision of professional services differs owing to commissioning and perhaps the fact that mental health is considered a specialism permeates provision.

When we explore the concept of crisis, we also need to consider risk and how this is perceived differently by individuals and hence this influences response. The work of Mary Douglas (1992), who defines risk 'as a representation' enables us to have a better understanding of risk and why professionals fear 'getting it wrong' or 'making poor decisions' when seeking to assist and support a person experiencing a crisis. In simplistic terms, exploring a blame culture helps us to understand why professionals may seek to control a situation and where possible, actively 'refer on', helping to manage and mitigate their manifested professional anxieties and burden. Furthermore, the work of Felton, Repper and Avis (2018) contributes to our understanding about viewing patients as 'risk objects', particularly following an adverse risk event. Risk connotations involving blame can be seen to transfer onto the professional in the form of tarnishing their reputation, suggesting clinicians interact less with mental health patients seen at risk (Felton, Repper and Avis, 2018).

As previously mentioned, professionals rarely work in isolation, and it is not solely their responsibility to respond and manage a person presenting in crisis and at risk. Variabilities in risk governance across national policy regimes exist and these differences are often transcultural-organisational in origin (Douglas, 1986). Rothstein (2006) suggests differing institutional risk management processes develop self-perpetuating rationales and these factors are shaped by, and impact upon, changing forms of trust relationships across society and the ever-evolving interplay between authority, transparency and genuineness (Alaszewski, 2003, 2015; Brown and Michael, 2002). It is therefore important that professionals are aware of and recognise their positionality but also be attentive to different sub-groups within political systems. Acknowledging how differing experiences and personal beliefs, together with perceptions of government and healthcare organisations/structures, shape the intersections and social constructs of society (including race, gender, class and ethnicity) may help to better understand the various approaches to risk (Finucane *et al.*, 2000).

Finding mutual ground

Seeking to locate equilibrium between the expertise of the professional and that of the service user, while employing core values surrounding care, is key to crisis management (Royal College of Psychiatrists, 2021). This involves authentic diplomacy (developing a genuine rapport through effective communication), collaboration (the professional, where possible, assumes a complementary role, works cooperatively with the service user, sharing responsibility for problem-solving and making decisions to formulate/carry out plans for patient care), and negotiation (discussion aimed at reaching an agreement which, in this context, may include reducing significant risk, possibly suicide) (Symanski-Tondora *et al.*, 2014). When discussing collaboration, it is important to consider and draw on co-production when working with service users experiencing a crisis, while recognising and acknowledging this may be impacted upon by mitigating circumstances, for example, mental capacity and distress (discussed in detail in Chapter 2); hence co-production, in its purest form, may not always be possible.

The aim of co-production is to create a 'third space' where the knowledge and expertise of the clinician, in conjunction with the experience of/from the service user, can be shared (Rose and Kalathil, 2019). As previously considered, this may not be possible for a range of reasons, however, it also raises questions surrounding attainability due to the hierarchy that exists within clinical practice, resulting in a power dynamic between clinicians and service users. Despite the clinician's best efforts to promote service user voice, it is inevitable that some service users experiencing a crisis and presenting at risk will not feel equitable because of the legal and safeguarding frameworks in place (Mello, 2014). Ultimately, the aim is to promote meaningful, relevant, and impactful change to enable recovery via an equal partnership dynamic between the helping professional and the individual experiencing crisis.

The spectrum model

Earlier sections of the chapter encouraged the reader to consider, reflect and develop an understanding of definitions surrounding crisis, recovery, and risk and this helpfully forms a useful foundation on which to enhance understanding of differing terminology from personal, professional and stakeholder perspectives. However, focusing solely on singular and/or rigid definitions of what a crisis is and how risk is perceived may complicate matters and create narrowed vision through a distorted lens. In assigning definitions, we create a 'false economy' which stalls thinking and insight, when actually considering there may be a series of stages a person travels through helps us to percolate ideas that can be discussed and conceptualised between service(s), service users and significant others, alongside sketching out alternative ways of perceiving and responding to crises.

The seminal work of Keyes (2002) outlines the interconnected nature of mental health and illness, which has become more commonly known and accepted as the mental health spectrum (Bell, 2021; Westerhof and Keyes, 2010). The spectrum model provides a way of understanding the stages, and if new to crisis intervention work/management, this might be constructive in helping you to understand, rather than being concerned with and restricted by, multiple, complex definitions. Drawing on the spectrum model helps to conceptualise what stage/level the service user is at and helpfully links to the discussions in Chapter 3 surrounding the stress vulnerability model. See Figure 1.1.

Figure 1.1 The mental health spectrum model

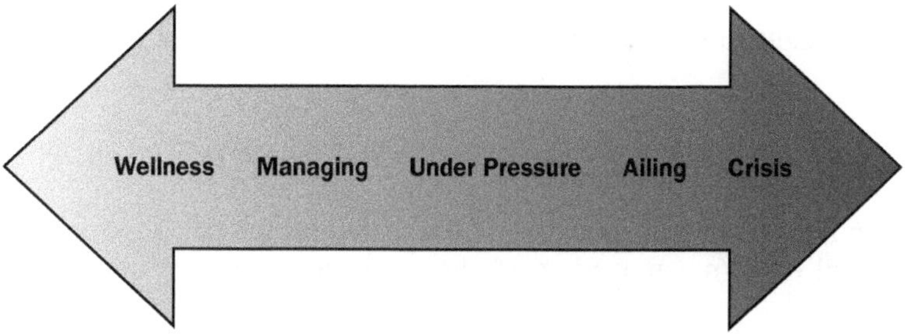

Wellness   Managing   Under Pressure   Ailing   Crisis

Source: Adapted from the Centre for Mental Health (2017), cited in Bell (2021).

At any one time, a person may be anywhere on the spectrum between 'wellness' and 'in crisis' and individuals move along the spectrum at different times, which reflects the fluidity of mental health (as seen in clinical and personal recovery). This may be understood by examining the mental health spectrum more closely. Under the 'ailing' descriptor, Bell (2021) suggests this involves mental health difficulties, causing a person significant distress and impairment. Should a person start to struggle and feel unwell, they may experience a period of compromised mental health and well-being, resulting in a crisis.

Individuals affected by a crisis event experience reactions that are fluid and changeable over time. Bourdieu (2019) describes the impact of habitus – interdependent relationships between people and the biophysical world – thus, individual characteristics, their understanding of the world, alongside relationships between each other can affect experiences and the interpretations of what a crisis might entail. Problem-solving skills acquired, for example, when growing up, and awareness of choices available as an adult, will influence perceptions of a crisis. The latter, as discussed in several chapters, can be shaped by burdensomeness; a sense that loved ones will have better lives without the person in them, thus increasing the risk of suicide. Hence the importance of considering human relationships, and if possible, connecting loved ones together as a support network, when providing crisis care.

The works of Horowitz (1986), Herman (1997) and latterly Yassen and Harvey (1998), suggest there are three primary phases of crisis reactions:

- *Acute Phase* – initial reactions in response to a traumatic event are usually physiological and psychological in nature.
- *Outward Adjustment Phase* – for some individuals, this phase may begin with a period of trauma followed by a period where the individual seeks/ attempts to gain some control by (re)engaging in routine, day-to-day activities.
- *Integration Phase* – the individual tries to make sense of what has happened and an important element of this is to try and resolve their sense of guilt and self-blame and start to make impactful changes to minimise the recurrence of the crisis.

To help us understand what characterises a crisis, let us consider the following stages:

A. The antecedent(s) or event(s) leading to the crisis perceived by the individual as threatening.
B. The individual feels unable to modify or reduce the impact of the precipitating stressful event(s), impacting on supporting relations, or abilities to seek support.
C. The experience of fear, tension and confusion escalates mental distress.
D. The individual experiences a high level of subjective discomfort.
E. The individual's state of equilibrium, i.e. abilities to cope, are compromised, resulting in an active state of crisis.
F. Experiencing a mental health crisis in which thoughts, emotions and behaviour may place the person in jeopardy of harming themselves and/or others and/or place the person at risk of some self-neglect.

It is useful here to further contemplate some links between the characteristics of a crisis and the mental health spectrum model, as a way of thinking about the underpinning knowledge surrounding crisis intervention work. This will enable a greater understanding through the use of the model and stages highlighted here, rather than being hindered by concerning ourselves with multiple definitions.

Drawing on the stages of the spectrum model as proposed by Bell (2021), a person is considered to be experiencing wellness when they are fulfilling their day-to-day living activities and thriving. At times, thriving may meander into 'managing', as day-to-day living is not without its challenges, but the flux between these two zones within the spectrum model are generally perceived as positive and the person is, in essence, well. The crux occurs when an individual starts to experience feeling 'under pressure' and this may become unmanageable for a range of reasons, including personal, social and/or environmental. Here we consider the person is situated at point A in the stages of a crisis; 'an antecedent and/or experience is perceived by the individual as threatening'. From this point, depending on an individual's coping mechanisms and the availability of or access to support, a person may start to spiral in terms of their ability to cope and manage the presenting cause (see stage B). Undoubtedly these factors will impact on mental well-being, causing mental distress and the person starts to 'ail' (see stages C and D). The combined elements across the initial stages (A–D) gather momentum, resulting in disequilibrium and feelings where a person is experiencing mental distress and lacks the ability to cope (stage E). For some, but not all, this results in a person experiencing a crisis (stage F) and may place the person in jeopardy of harming themselves or others and being placed at risk of self-neglect.

Conclusion

This chapter has considered the complex terrain surrounding defining and understanding the term 'crisis' and, in doing so, has sought to explore and explain commonly used terminology when working with and supporting a person experiencing a mental health crisis. What is not in doubt is that no single definition will suffice, nor will it capture the complex concepts which require a deeper awareness and understanding central to supporting crisis intervention care.

Concepts surrounding personal and clinical recovery were explored and how recovery is situated within crisis intervention and management work was explained. Notions of risk were also explored and help us to situate interconnected concepts relating to the experience of a crisis and an individual's personal journey of recovery. This, in conjunction with a relatively brief overview and exploration of what constitutes a crisis and the mental health spectrum model, enables readers, whether new to crisis work or a seasoned professional, to (re)visit their understandings of what a crisis is, and what crisis work might entail.

It is important for all helping professionals and other stakeholders involved in helping a person in crisis to develop a sense of solidarity and promote co-production, enabling individuals and their families/carers to be empowered, thus fostering an equitable shared sense of responsibility and giving voice to patients to influence the structures, boundaries and provision of care. While mental health practitioners may be perceived as providing specialist interventions, it is important that all helping professionals recognise, value and respond to the spectrum of mental health crisis in a sensitive and person-centred way, engaging in helpful interprofessional dialogue and confidently signposting. Overall, this chapter has created the conceptual foundations to underpin the following chapters, enabling readers to understand, develop and extend their roles when working with a person experiencing a crisis.

Further reading

- **Co-production:**
  Peter, S. and Schulz, G. (2018) 'I-as-We': Powerful boundaries within the field of mental health coproduction. *International Journal of Mental Health Nursing*, 27(4), 1292–1300.
- **King's Fund, *Joined Up Listening*:**
  https://www.kingsfund.org.uk/publications/joined-up-listening-integrated-care-and-patient-insight
- **Mental Health Network, Briefing Paper:** https://www.nhsconfed.org/~/media/Confederation/Files/Publications/Documents/mental-health-crisis-care.PDF
- **NHS England, Integrated Care Recommendations:** https://www.england.nhs.uk/integratedcare/
- **Personal recovery:**
  Leamy, M., Bird, V., Le Boutillier, C., Williams, J. and Slade, M. (2011) Conceptual framework for personal recovery in mental health: Systematic review and narrative synthesis. *British Journal of Psychiatry*, 199, 445–452.
- **Promoting recovery through care planning:**
  Hall, A., Wren, M. and Kirby, S.D. (2013) *Care Planning in Mental Health: Promoting Recovery*, 2nd edn. Chichester: Wiley Blackwell.
- **Risk:**
  Lupton, D. (2013) *Risk (Key Ideas)*, 2nd edn. London: Routledge.

References

Alaszewski, A. (2003) Risk, trust and health. *Health, Risk and Society*, 5(3), 235–239.
Alaszewski, A. (2015) Anthropology and risk: Insights into uncertainty, danger and blame from other cultures: A review essay. *Health, Risk and Society*, 17(3–4), 205–225.

Anthony, W.A. (1993) Recovery from mental illness: The guiding vision of the mental health service system in the 1990s. *Innovations and Research in Clinical Services, Community Support, and Rehabilitation*, 2, 17–24.

Barber, M.E. (2012) Recovery as the new medical model for psychiatry. *Psychiatric Services*, 63(3), 277–279.

Bell, A. (2021) Mental health for all: Working across the spectrum. Blog. Centre for Mental Health. Available at: https://www.centreformentalhealth.org.uk/blogs/mental-health-all-working-across-spectrum (accessed 29 May 2021).

Bourdieu, P. (2019) *Habitus and Field: General Sociology*, vol. 2: *(1982–1983)*. Cambridge: Polity Press.

Brown, B. (2021) Responsibilization and recovery: Shifting responsibilities on the journey through mental health care to social engagement. *Social Theory and Health*, 19(1), 92–109.

Brown, N. and Michael, M. (2002) From authority to authenticity: The changing governance of biotechnology. *Health, Risk and Society*, 4(3), 259–272.

Caplan, G. (1964) *Principles of Preventive Psychiatry*. New York: Basic Books.

Centre for Mental Health (2021) Updated: Centre for Mental Health responds to the Serenity Integrated Mentoring (SIM) model. Available at: https://www.centreformentalhealth.org.uk/news/updated-centre-mental-health-responds-serenity-integrated-mentoring-sim-model (accessed 27 June 2021).

Cook, A. (2019) Taking a holistic approach to acute mental health crisis. *Journal of Paramedic Practice: The Clinical Monthly for Emergency Care Professionals*, 11(10), 426–432.

CQC (Care Quality Commission) (2015) Right here, right now: People's experiences of help, care and support during a mental health crisis. Available at: https://www.cqc.org.uk/sites/default/files/20150630_righthere_mhcrisiscare_full.pdf (accessed 29 May 2021).

CQC (Care Quality Commission) (2020) Community Mental Health Survey: Statistical Release. Available at: https://www.cqc.org.uk/sites/default/files/20201124_cmh20_statisticalrelease.pdf (accessed 3 January 2021).

Deegan, P.E. (1988) Recovery: The lived experience of rehabilitation. *Psychosocial Rehabilitation Journal*, 11, 11–19.

Deering, K., Pawson, C., Summers, N. and Williams, J. (2019) Patient perspectives of helpful risk management practices within mental health services. A mixed studies systematic review of primary research. *Journal of Psychiatric and Mental Health Nursing*, 26(5–6), 185–197.

Deering, K., Williams, J., Stayner, K. and Pawson, C. (2021) Giving a voice to patient experiences through the insights of pragmatism. *Nursing Philosophy*, 22(1), 1–9.

Department of Health (2004) *The Ten Essential Shared Capabilities: A Framework for the Whole Health and Social Care Workforce*. London: Department of Health.

Douglas, M. (1986) *How Institutions Think*. New York: Syracuse University Press.

Douglas, M. (1992) *Risk and Blame: Essays in Cultural Theory*. New York: Routledge.

Felton, A., Repper, J. and Avis, M. (2018) The construction of people with mental health problem as risk objects: Findings of a case study review. *Journal of Psychiatric and Mental Health Nursing*, 25(9–10), 558–568.

Finucane, M., Slovic, P., Mertz, C., Flynn, J. and Satterfield, T. (2000) Gender, race, and perceived risk: The 'white male' effect. *Health, Risk and Society*, 2(2), 159–172.

Greene, G., Lee, M., Trask, R. and Rheinscheld, J. (2000) How to work with clients' strengths in crisis intervention. In A.R. Roberts (ed.) *Crisis Intervention Handbook: Assessment, Treatment and Research*. Oxford: Oxford University Press, pp. 31–55.

Gregory, M.J. and Thompson, A. (2013) From here to recovery: One service user's journey through a mental health crisis: Some reflections on experience, policy and practice. *Journal of Social Work Practice*, 27(4), 455–470.

Heath, R.L. (2006) Best practices in crisis communication: Evolution of practice through research. *Journal of Applied Communication Research*, 34(3), 245–248.

Herman, J.L. (1997) *Trauma and Recovery*. New York: Basic Books.

Horowitz, M.J. (1986) Stress-response syndromes: A review of posttraumatic and adjustment disorders. *Hospital and Community Psychiatry*, 37(3), 241–249.

James, R.K. and Gilliland, B.E. (2005) *Crisis Intervention Strategies*. Belmont, CA: Thomson.

Keyes, C.L.M. (2002) The mental health continuum: From languishing to flourishing in life. *Journal of Health and Social Behavior*, 43(2), 207–222.

Lavoie, J.A.A. (2018) Relative invisibility: An integrative review of carers' lived experiences of a family member's emergency mental health crisis. *Social Work in Mental Health*, 16(5), 601–626.

Lloyd-Evans, B. and Johnson, F. (2014) Crisis resolution teams: How are they performing? *Mental Health Today*. Available at: https://pubmed.ncbi.nlm.nih.gov/32517530/ (accessed 28 June 2021).

Mello, P.A. (2014) A comparative analysis of constitutional and political restrictions on the use of force. Available at: https://papers.ssrn.com/sol3/papers.cfm?abstract_id=2477716 (accessed 28 June 2021).

Mind (2014) Mental health services 'cut by 8 per cent'. Available at: https://www.mind.org.uk/news-campaigns/news/mental-health-services-cut-by-8-per-cent/ (accessed 28 June 2021).

Mind (2020) Data analysis by Mind has revealed that more people have experienced a mental health crisis during the coronavirus pandemic than ever previously. Available at: https://www.mind.org.uk/news-campaigns/news/mind-warns-of-second-pandemic-as-it-reveals-more-people-in-mental-health-crisis-than-ever-recorded-and-helpline-calls-soar/ (accessed 28 June 2021).

Molodynski, A., McLellan, A., Craig, T. and Bhugra, D. (2020) What does COVID mean for UK mental health care? *International Journal of Social Psychiatry*. Available at: https://journals.sagepub.com/doi/full/10.1177/0020764020932592 (accessed 28 June 2021).

Morant, N., Lloyd-Evans, B., Lamb, D., Fullarton, K., Brown, E., Paterson, B., Istead, H., Kelly, K., Hindle, D., … and CORE Service User and Carer Working Groups (2017) Crisis resolution and home treatment: Stakeholders' views on critical ingredients and implementation in England. *BMC Psychiatry*, 17(1), 1–13.

NICE (National Institute for Clinical Excellence) (2011) *Improving Your Experience of Mental Health Services in the NHS*. Available at: https://www.nice.org.uk/guidance/cg136/resources/improving-your-experience-of-mental-health-services-in-the-nhs-pdf-239823925189 (accessed 28 June 2021).

NICE (National Institute for Clinical Excellence) (2016) *Achieving Better Access to 24/7 Urgent and Emergency Mental Health Care – Part 2: Implementing the Evidence-based Treatment Pathway for Urgent and Emergency Liaison Mental Health Services for Adults and Older Adults – Guidance*. Available at: https://www.nice.org.uk/guidance/ng10/resources/evidencebased-treatment-pathway-for-urgent-and-emergency-liaison-mental-health-services-for-adults-and-older-adults-guidance-pdf-4362198589 (accessed 28 June 2021).

O'Keeffe, D., Sheridan, A., Kelly, A., Doyle, R., Madigan, K., Lawlor, E. and Clarke, M. (2018) Recovery in the real world: Service user experiences of mental health service use and recommendations for change 20 years on from a first episode psychosis. *Administration and Policy in Mental Health and Mental Health Services Research,* 45(4), 635–648.

Oxford English Dictionary (2021) Crisis. Available at: https://www.oed.com/view/ Entry/44539?redirectedFrom=crisis#eid (accessed 28 June 2021).

Paton, F., Wright, K., Ayre, N., Dare, C., Johnson, S., Lloyd-Evans, B., Simpson, A., Webber, M. and Meader, N. (2016) Improving outcomes for people in mental health crisis: A rapid synthesis of the evidence for available models of care. *Health Technology Assessment,* 20(3), 1–162.

Peterson, C. and Seligman, M.E.P. (2004) *Character Strengths and Virtues: A Handbook of Classification.* Oxford: Oxford University Press.

Pulvirenti, M., McMillan, J. and Lawn, S. (2014) Empowerment, patient-centred care and self-management. *Health Expectations: An International Journal of Public Participation in Health Care and Health Policy,* 17(3), 303–310.

RCP (Royal College of Psychiatrists) (2021) Co-production values and principles in liaison person-centred assessment and beyond. Available from: https://www.rcpsych. ac.uk/docs/default-source/improving-care/ccqi/quality-networks/psychiatric-liaison-services-plan/steph-using-co-production-values.pdf?sfvrsn=96e1c1bf_2 (accessed 18 June 2021).

Repper, J. and Perkins, R. (2003) *Social Inclusion and Recovery: A Model for Mental Health Practice.* London: Bailliere Tindall.

Roberts, A.R. and Ottens, A.J. (2005) The seven-stage crisis intervention model: A road map to goal attainment, problem solving, and crisis resolution. *Brief Treatment and Crisis Intervention,* 5(4), 329–339.

Rose, D. and Kalathil, J. (2019) Power, privilege and knowledge: The untenable promise of co-production in mental 'health'. *Frontiers in Sociology.* Available at: https://www. frontiersin.org/articles/10.3389/fsoc.2019.00057/full (accessed 28 June 2021).

Rothstein, H. (2006) The institutional origins of risk: A new agenda for risk research. *Health, Risk and Society,* 8(3), 215–221.

Roy, A. and Buchanan, J. (2016) The paradoxes of recovery policy: Exploring the impact of austerity and responsibilisation for the citizenship claims of people with drug problems. *Social Policy and Administration,* 50(3), 398–413.

Ruggeri, M. and Tansella, M. (2012) People-centred mental health care. The interplay between the individual perspective and the broader health care context. *Epidemiology and Psychiatric Sciences,* 21(2), 125–129.

Slade, M. (2009) *Personal Recovery and Mental Illness: A Guide for Mental Health Professionals.* Cambridge: Cambridge University Press.

Slade, M., Amering, M., Farkas, M., Hamilton, B., O'Hagan, M., Panther, G., Perkins, R., Shepherd, G., … and Whitley, R. (2014) Uses and abuses of recovery: Implementing recovery-oriented practices in mental health systems. *World Psychiatry,* 13(1), 12–20.

Storm, M. and Edwards, A. (2013) Models of user involvement in the mental health context: Intentions and implementation challenges. *Psychiatric Quarterly,* 84(3), 313–327.

Sukut, O. and Ayhan Balik, C.H. (2021) The impact of COVID-19 pandemic on people with severe mental illness. *Perspectives in Psychiatric Care,* 57(2), 953–956.

Symanski-Tondora, J., Miller, R., Slade, M. and Davidson, L. (2014) *Partnering for Recovery in Mental Health.* Chichester: Wiley-Blackwell.

Tse, S., Tsoi, E.W., Hamilton, B., O'Hagan, M., Shepherd, G., Slade, M., Whitley, R. and Petrakis, M. (2016) Uses of strength-based interventions for people with serious mental illness: A critical review. *International Journal of Social Psychiatry*, 62(3), 281–291.

Tse, S., Yuen, W.W.Y., Murray, G., Davidson, L., Lai, Q. and Kan, A. (2019) Combining technical and expert-by-experience knowledge in the quest for personal recovery from bipolar disorder: A qualitative study. *BMC Psychiatry*, 19(1), 1–12.

Westerhof, G.J. and Keyes, C.LM. (2010) Mental illness and mental health: The two conti-nua model across the lifespan. *Journal of Adult Development*, 17(2), 110–119.

Yassen, J. and Harvey, M.R. (1998) Crisis assessment and interventions with victims of violence. In P.M. Kleespies (ed.) *Emergencies in Mental Health Practice*. New York: Guilford Press, pp. 117–143.

2 | Mental health crises in an emergency department

Andy Hill and Amy Manley

Introduction

In *A History of Self-Harm in Britain* (Millard, 2015), the case of Laura Ashby is outlined. Ashby cuts her throat and is brought to the general hospital by the police. Records show a dispute between the hospital matron and police officer concerning who should take responsibility for ensuring Ashby's safety while she receives treatment. The year is 1914. For those working in an emergency department (ED) today, this is likely to resonate. By necessity, the ED is the most readily accessible part of the NHS (National Health Service) where members of the public can self-present and other services can direct patients. Such accessibility provides unique challenges with respect to mental health crises.

In this chapter, we provide guidance on the assessment and management of mental health crises in ED. This includes the medico-legal aspects of treatment and the overlap between physical and mental health, both of which can be crucial considerations in ED. We focus on three common presentations – deliberate self-harm (DSH), suicidality, and acute psychosis – which are associated with risk and tend to generate anxiety. Although we hope that the material provided in this chapter will be of benefit to specialists in mental health, particularly the focus on assessment, it is primarily aimed at medical and nursing staff in ED.

Psychiatric attendances to emergency departments

Hospital episode statistics report that three times more people attended EDs in England with a primary mental health problem in 2019–2020, compared to a decade earlier (NHS Digital, 2020). Such presentations range from the relatively straightforward, for example, panic attacks and minor acts of self-harm, to complex co-morbidity. With respect to the latter, consider case study 2.1.

Case study 2.1 Bernadette

Bernadette is a 27-year-old who has self-presented to ED for the fifth time in two weeks. As with the previous presentations, she has made lacerations to her legs and arms. These lacerations appear more extensive and deeper on each presentation. On this occasion, she has also taken a paracetamol overdose. Bernadette reports a long history of substance misuse, depression and anxiety. Her mood has deteriorated in the last few weeks following a relationship breakdown. She also reports a history of voice hearing. In recent days, the voices have become more frequent and intense. Last night, they instructed her to kill herself and hence she overdosed. Bernadette is usually difficult to engage with, sometimes withdrawn, at other times hostile. While being sutured, she informs the examining doctor that she might not stay for treatment for the overdose if it is required.

Bernadette's case highlights some of the challenges for ED staff. How best to respond to someone who is attending frequently with self-harm? Is the voice hearing indicative of acute psychosis and, if so, how might this affect the management of Bernadette in ED? If she does require treatment for the overdose and refuses, should she be forcibly treated?

The role of liaison psychiatry

Complex presentations, like Bernadette's, should be referred for specialist psychiatric assessments. Liaison psychiatry services based in the general hospital work alongside ED clinicians to collect information, conduct assessments, and develop safe and effective management plans (House and Akagi, 2012). If a patient attending ED is under the care of a mental health team, it is preferable for a clinician from that team to conduct the assessment, however, this is usually impractical. In such cases, the assessment is usually conducted by the liaison team, which reduces waiting times. Liaison teams also provide expertise in the overlap between mental and physical health (Leigh, 2015). The majority of hospitals have such a service but fewer than half operate 24 hours a day (Walker *et al.*, 2018). The importance of offering a 24-hour service is highlighted by the fact that the majority of psychiatric ED attendances occur between 22:00 and 07:00 (NHS England, National Collaborating Centre for Mental Health, and National Institute for Clinical Excellence (NICE), 2016). During these hours, specialist assessment may instead be provided by off-site mental health teams such as crisis services, although such provision can be limited. Irrespective of which service conducts the specialist assessment, it should be emphasised that the overnight discharge of patients in crisis carries additional risks and could lead to more restrictive practices compared to seeing a patient after a period of reflection.

The challenges to the delivery of psychiatric care in the ED

Environmental challenges

The design of an ED is generally not conducive to caring for patients experiencing a mental health crisis. Care is delivered in open cubicles for observation purposes and easy access to equipment; however, these aspects of the physical environment also pose challenges when managing patients who are behaviourally disturbed. Equipment in the environment could be used to self-harm. The ease of access to bed spaces can lead to interference with the care of other patients. The proximity to other patients who have acute medical needs can be distressing, while noise and activity levels in treatment areas can add to distress. For acutely psychotic individuals, over-stimulating environments can aggravate hallucinations and delusional beliefs. Patients with persecutory ideas may misinterpret routine nursing and medical interventions, increasing distress and hostility. Moreover, the noise levels combined with lack of privacy make it difficult to engage in sensitive and lengthy conversations concerning mental health problems.

Waiting areas can also be challenging places. Patients who self-present to the ED are, on arrival, required to give personal details to a receptionist in what is often a crowded waiting room. Moreover, the waiting room can often feel an unsafe place to be. For those brought in by ambulance at busy times, there is the possibility of having to wait for a prolonged period either in the ambulance or in a queue in a corridor, or both, because of limited space in the department.

Waiting times and multiple assessments

Waiting for a prolonged period in an ambulance queue or a noisy crowded waiting area can cause frustration and exacerbate distress. Another source of potential frustration and distress is the number of times patients are expected to tell their story (Koning, McNaught and Tuffin, 2018). At a minimum, this usually includes the receptionist, the triage nurse and ED staff. Patients often face delays between assessments, particularly if they have no physical health needs. If a specialist mental health assessment is required, there is likely to be a further delay. Moreover, this involves a further telling of the story. A small number of patients will require additional psychiatric assessments to determine if detention under the Mental Health Act (1983) is necessary. This will result in a further delay while the relevant staff are assembled from outside the hospital. It also requires yet another telling of the story. Because of increasing shortages of beds in psychiatric hospitals, those patients who are detained can sometimes be required to wait in the ED for days rather than hours.

Emotionally challenging patients and the impact on staff

The primary function of an ED is to provide rapid assessment and treatment of people with acute physical health problems, some of which are life-threatening and, therefore, require urgent medical intervention. Because of the emphasis on medical intervention, many ED clinicians report feeling 'out of their comfort zone' when delivering care to patients with mental health problems. Supporting patients in distress is emotionally demanding and behavioural disturbance can be frightening and stressful. Staff who witness patients further harming themselves in ED can feel traumatised and experience a sense of failure about not having prevented it. Anxiety is a common emotional response to those experiencing a mental health crisis. In part, this arises out of concerns about being insufficiently skilled and experienced. This is particularly so with respect to managing risk of suicide. In such cases, there is usually a range of concerns, including: 'What should I say or ask? Will what I say and ask make things worse? What should I do if this person wants to leave?' Some patients elicit feelings of fear, powerlessness, ambivalence and emotional exhaustion, which can contribute to negative attitudes and lack of empathy among clinicians (Rayner, Blackburn, Edward, Stephenson and Ousey, 2019; Woollaston and Hixenbaugh, 2008).

Patients who are objecting to care are often the most emotionally challenging. This sometimes arises because patients are frightened and/or angry, which is particularly common among the minority of patients who have been coercively brought to ED (for example, having been detained by the police). At times, such patients may become aggressive or violent, or attempt to abscond. On the occasions when it is necessary to physically restrain a patient, staff do so without the practical resources or legislative power of a specifically designed psychiatric hospital. Unlike those staff working in a psychiatric hospital, ED staff have only limited Prevention and Management of Violence and Aggression (PMVA) training. Although assistance can be sought from hospital security, this is a limited resource. The police are often unable to attend. Because patients in ED are not deemed to be admitted to the hospital, there is no recourse to the Mental Health Act. Therefore, in cases where restraint and/or rapid tranquillisation is required, clinicians are often forced to make complex 'on the spot' capacity decisions, sometimes with little knowledge about the patient. Moreover, the restraint of a patient requires the diversion of a significant number of already busy staff from the care of other patients, most of whom have acute medical needs.

There are two other forms of objecting to care that are particularly emotionally challenging. First, from those whose expectations did not align well with the outcome of mental health assessments. For example, patients with psychosis, who disagree that they are ill, can find the decision to detain them under the Mental Health Act extremely distressing, which may result in aggression and/or absconding. Patients who have harmed themselves or feel suicidal, and their families, often come to ED with the expectation of a psychiatric admission and feel rejected and angry when community care is advised. In such cases, patients sometimes refuse to leave, harm themselves in the department, or state that they will leave and complete suicide. Second, objecting to care can take the form of treatment refusal. This is particularly challenging and stressful when the treatment required is potentially life-saving, for example, following a paracetamol overdose.

Interprofessional disagreements

There are occasions when the repeated presentation to the ED of someone in crisis can generate conflict between professionals. Consider case study 2.2.

Case study 2.2   Aisha

Aisha is an 18-year-old non-binary person who, as a child, was a victim of recurrent sexual abuse by their stepfather. They have a long history of self-harm, and their arms show scars at various stages of healing. More recently, they have started to cut their legs and have presented to the ED three times in the last week, requiring sutures. Aisha is not currently under the care of mental health services. They had one admission to a psychiatric hospital last year where their self-harm increased. From there, Aisha was discharged to the community mental health team but did not engage and was discharged back to the General Practitioner (GP), who is concerned about the escalating self-harm but feels powerless to help. Aisha is warm and friendly towards most of the ED staff, expressing gratitude for the care received. The frustrated ED doctor thinks that Aisha should be sectioned to get 'proper help' and stop the presentations to the ED. The crisis team disagree and maintain that Aisha should continue to be managed by the GP.

In such cases, ED clinicians may blame other individuals or teams for the patient's presentation, believing that 'if only they did their job' the patient would not harm themselves. Criticism of others is a natural response to feeling powerless, however, it might be the case that Aisha only engages with health professionals at times of acute distress, for example, after Aisha has self-harmed. If so, there is a risk of 'splitting' – the generation of polarised opinions – between different teams. This risk is accentuated if the patient idolises and demonises different professionals. For example, being told 'you're the first clinician who has understood me, my psychiatrist never listens' is flattering and may encourage one to cross the usual boundaries for the patient. 'Splitting' can also occur within teams. In Aisha's case, some staff may feel resentful about their repeat attendances, while others are highly concerned. Such polarised responses can impair team functioning, including the ability to support each other (Green, 2018).

Interpersonal challenges and the patient experience

Returning to the case of Bernadette described in case study 2.1, consider what she might think as she contemplates attending the ED:

> I know I need help now, but I hate going there. The waiting room is usually full and half the people in there are drunk. It's so noisy. The voice I hear has

come back, and that, combined with all the noise, makes it overwhelming. The worst part is having to stand there telling the receptionist that I have hurt myself in front of everyone. I know they're judging me. I feel so self-conscious. I always have to wait ages to be seen and when I do get seen, some staff aren't very nice. I know some of them think I'm a time-waster. Some of the others look really anxious and don't seem to know what to say. I'll get myself stitched up, but I'll probably take my chances with the overdose. The last thing I need is a night in there with all those machines beeping and people screaming and shouting.

Bernadette's concerns reflect some of the challenges outlined above, for example, the noisy environment and prolonged waiting times. She also highlights concerns about the way in which she might be perceived and treated by staff. Many people attending ED with mental health problems share these concerns. For some, this will be based on previous negative experiences in which they felt judged, misunderstood, or received sub-optimal care. Even within the last 20 years there have been reports of people with self-inflicted lacerations being sutured without anaesthetic (National Collaborating Centre for Mental Health UK, 2004). Such experiences can echo abuse histories and discourage more productive ways to seek help. Even at first attendance, the stigma associated with mental health problems can lead people to assume that they will be perceived as a time-waster, reinforcing feelings of worthlessness and hopelessness. One of Bernadette's concerns is that some of the staff appear anxious and do not know what to say to her. It is worth noting that difficult feelings arising in clinicians often closely mirror the emotional state of the patient themselves, who is unable to communicate their experience through other means. If clinicians deal with their own difficult feelings by being critical, emotionally distant, or ambivalent, it increases the likelihood of the patient feeling rejected.

Responding to the challenges

In this section we provide some suggestions for how to respond to the challenges outlined above. The discussion concerning how to improve the patient experience with respect to the interpersonal dimension of care requires more detail and is the subject of the section 'Interpersonal skills'. A discussion of how to respond to treatment refusal is the subject of the section 'Treatment refusal and the legal framework for care'.

Environmental challenges

- *Lack of privacy*: Although the need to provide optimal physical care will often trump concerns about privacy in the ED, clinicians should demonstrate sensitivity with respect to this issue. This should include acknowledging with the patient the lack of privacy and, if possible, having discussions about particularly sensitive issues, for example, suicide and domestic violence in a more private area. It is essential that the ED provides assessment rooms to facilitate privacy, however, these must meet safety standards.

- *Noise and over-stimulation*: Staff should be aware of the detrimental effects of excessive noise and over-stimulation, particularly with respect to acutely psychotic patients. The use of side rooms, if available, in conjunction with allocating a 1:1 specialist nurse is likely to reduce both noise and stimulation, and the risk of absconding and behavioural disturbance.

Waiting times and multiple assessments

Options for improving the response times of on-site liaison psychiatry teams:

- *Setting target response times* for patients in crisis to be seen.
- *Parallel triage*: A mental health specialist conducts triage assessments with the triage nurse. This informs treatment while in the ED and can facilitate earlier psychosocial assessment.
- *Direct referrals to liaison psychiatry*: Medically fit patients may be referred directly to psychiatry at point of triage, thus reducing the need for the patient to tell their story to an ED doctor or emergency nurse practitioner (ENP). This requires good joint working due to the diagnostic overlap between psychiatric and physical symptoms. It is less suitable for older adults, those with learning or cognitive difficulties, and people unknown to psychiatric services, where diagnostic uncertainty is common.
- *Parallel assessment and treatment*: If a patient can engage appropriately with the consultation, psychiatric assessments can be safely completed before the patient is declared 'medically fit', for example, while a patient is treated for paracetamol overdose. However, if the outcome is likely to change with improved physical health, later assessment or reassessment may be needed.
- *Information provision*: Consider providing information about the ED experience, local services, and coping mechanisms at reception or in the waiting room. This ensures patients have this information, should they choose to leave. It also helps manage expectations, highlights ways to cope with the environment (for example, digital relaxation apps), and promotes hopefulness by signposting services to help.

Options for improving the response times of external teams:

- *Developing strong working relationships between hospital managers, ED staff, ED team, and crisis teams*. This should include a forum to meet and discuss problematic situations, engage in problem-solving, and develop pathways that reduce unnecessary multiple assessments for patients attending the ED.

- *Developing an agreed escalation policy when delays occur*, for example, waiting for a Mental Health Act assessment or a bed in a psychiatric hospital.
- *Clear monitoring of key performance indicators* such as delays to assessments can inform service provision and support longer-term strategy (this should also apply to on-site teams).

Emotionally challenging patients and the impact on staff

Disturbed behaviour

Contrary to popular belief, the majority of violence among people with mental health problems is explained by confounding factors such as alcohol, drug use and socio-economic deprivation (Elbogen and Johnson, 2009). Below are some management strategies for what to do when disturbed behaviour arises:

- *Documentation and collateral information*: Regardless of the presence of mental disorder, the strongest predictor of future risk of aggression is past behaviour. Therefore, robust documentation and alert systems are valuable to identify patients with a history of aggression who may pose risks to staff so measures can be taken to ensure staff safety, while not adversely affecting the patient's care.
- *Assessment rooms*: Psychiatric assessments take place in a suitable room (for example, with an observation panel and fitted with an alarm) as detailed by the Psychiatric Liaison Accreditation Network (PLAN) (RCP, 2020).
- *Verbal de-escalation*: This includes relocating to a low stimuli area, maintaining a safe distance, the use of non-threatening body language and a calm tone of voice. Staff should listen to the patient's concerns, empathise, establish a rapport and negotiate a solution.
- *The use of medication*: If verbal de-escalation is insufficient, some patients may benefit from oral medication to reduce their distress. Where rapid tranquillisation is needed, this should follow NICE (2015) (or other relevant local) guidance unless there is a clear rationale for deviating from the guidance, in which case this should involve senior input, discussion with the patient or their advocates, where feasible, and relevant speciality teams, for example, psychiatry and anaesthetics. Although ED has some disadvantages for psychiatric care, it does have rapid access to baseline investigations (bloods and electrocardiogram (ECG)), treatment for potential side effects (for example, dystonia), and expert colleagues (for example, anaesthetists). The advice of anaesthetic colleagues is particularly valuable when considering the risks, benefits and practicalities of sedation to facilitate treatment or investigation. Covert medication under an appropriate legal framework is also an option, although this is rare, given the relatively short time a patient will spend in the ED.
- *Physical restraint*: This should always be a last resort. The guiding principles are that restraint is both necessary and proportionate. Ideally, it should be carried out by a minimum of three staff who have been trained in PMVA.

In view of the amount of aggression and violence in the ED, consideration should be given to improving staff training.

Dissatisfaction with the outcome of assessments:

- It is important to manage expectations from the outset. Be realistic and do not make promises, for example, 'I'm sure the Liaison Psychiatry team will sort this out.' Say instead: 'It might be helpful for you to have an assessment with the Liaison Psychiatry team, and you can think about some of these problems together.' For patients who are already under the care of community mental health teams, it is unlikely that significant changes to their management will be made in the ED.
- Good interpersonal skills are vital when explaining the rationale for treatment decisions.

Supporting staff

Senior endorsement of strategies to support staff in managing distressing clinical encounters is vital to their success. The following can be helpful:

- Debriefing with senior clinicians after specific incidents such as aggression.
- Discussion of complex and challenging presentations with liaison psychiatry input.
- Ensuring there is space and opportunity for informal discussion and debrief.
- Education and training programmes covering relevant psychiatric topics, for example, self-harm, suicide, legal frameworks, and rapid tranquillisation.
- Inclusion of mental health in induction of new staff.

Interprofessional disagreements

Managing divided opinions

It is important that all staff have an opportunity to raise concerns about a patient's care, both within their own team and more widely. However, it is important to emphasise that in complex cases it is unusual that a single person or team could make all the difference. In such cases, where attachment difficulties are evident, successful care requires a consistent, planned approach. The following strategies can reduce 'splitting' within and between teams:

- Recognising and discussing divided opinions.
- Hearing and respecting other professionals' concerns, as opposed to responding defensively.
- Recognising the complexity of clinical decisions and respecting different professionals' roles.

- Providing clear rationales for clinical decisions.
- Being open to the possibility that a patient's presentation may have changed since your assessment and that this may have had implications for their care.
- Supporting the patient in discussing their concerns with the team they are criticising (or relevant complaints service, if appropriate) rather than colluding in the criticism. For example, 'I can see you are upset about that outcome, but I don't know much about the housing system, do you think it would be helpful to speak to your social worker directly?'

A system-wide approach

When services are overstretched, it is easy to overlook the impact that clinical decisions may have on other areas of the health system. For example, the decision of a GP to prescribe medications that are later used to overdose, or demand admission for a patient who has previously responded poorly to such an intervention. System-wide care can be facilitated by doing the following:

- Consideration of a team's decisions on other areas of the patient's 'system' (professional and personal supports) and discussion with teams which may be impacted.
- Multi-disciplinary meetings involving multiple agencies (including emergency care providers) involved in patient care increase buy-in and ensure consistent care.
- Care plans that consider potential likely consequences of clinical decisions, for example, increased ED or GP attendance following community team discharge.

Interpersonal skills

Many of the responses to the challenges highlighted above emphasise the need for good interpersonal skills with both patients and other professionals. With respect to patient care, this is particularly important because it not only has a significant impact on the patient experience but also the interpersonal dimension of caring for someone experiencing a mental health crisis is arguably the one that is most within the clinician's control. Good interpersonal skills are an integral part of engagement with patients. Engagement can be understood as the process of establishing a mutually trusting and respectful helping relationship (Miller and Rollnick, 2013). It is essential that ED clinicians do not regard engagement as the sole domain of mental health specialists. Even with relatively brief interactions, for example, a triage assessment, good engagement skills can greatly improve the patient experience. Moreover, such skills enhance assessments by enabling the clinician to gain a more accurate understanding of the patient's situation, including the level of risk. In this section, we illustrate the value of good engagement skills with respect to both suicidal (case study 2.3) and acutely psychotic patients (case study 2.4).

Talking with a patient contemplating suicide

Case study 2.3   David

David is a 54-year-old man who has somewhat reluctantly been brought to ED by a friend after disclosing that he is having thoughts about hanging himself. His friend is unable to wait with him. On arrival, he appears distressed and agitated. He was treated for an episode of depression in his thirties, during which he made an attempt to hang himself. He has been feeling 'desperate' for a month since being made redundant from his job as an accountant, which he has had for more than 20 years. Following this, his relationship has ended. After registering at reception, 30 minutes later he sees the triage nurse.

Compare the two ways in which the triage nurse engages with David in Table 2.1.

Table 2.1 Principles for supporting people with behavioural disturbance

A Poor engagement	B Good engagement
N: Why have you come here today? D: Because I feel suicidal.	N: Tell me what's brought you to an Emergency Department today. D: Because I feel suicidal.
N: Have you done anything to yourself? D: No. N: Okay, and do you have any problems with your physical health? D: No, I don't think so.	N: I'm sorry to hear that. It sounds really tough. Tell me a bit more about what's been happening recently. D: Everything's going wrong. I've lost my job and now my wife has walked out. In the last couple of weeks I've felt really depressed and I'm not sure there's much point in carrying on.
N: Okay, but I need to take your blood pressure, pulse, and temperature. D: Alright.	N: So, there's been a lot of really difficult things happening, which have started to affect your mood, and made you think about whether life is worth living. D: Yeah, that's about it.
N: After I've done that, I need to take some more details about why you came today. D: Alright.	N: I know this can be really difficult to talk about, but I need to check if you have tried to kill yourself recently. D: I came close to hanging myself last night.

(Continued)

Table 2.1   (Continued)

A Poor engagement	B Good engagement
N: So, why do you feel like killing yourself? D: Everything's going wrong. N: Like what? D: I've lost my job. N: Anything else? D: My marriage is over. N: Has anything else happened? D: No. N: Okay, so it's important that you see the mental health team and you can tell them all about it. D: I suppose I should. N: Are you having any thoughts about killing yourself now? D: I don't know. The thoughts come and go. N: So, if I put you back in the waiting room do you think you could act on these thoughts? D: I guess not. N: Okay, I'll put you back in the waiting room and make a referral to the mental health team. I'm sorry but I don't know how long it will take. D: Alright.	N: I'm really glad you didn't. You seem quite distressed now. How do you feel about seeing one of the mental health specialists here? D: That's why my friend brought me. I suppose I should. N: You sound a bit reluctant. D: Yeah, I just can't get these thoughts about hanging out of my head. N: How safe do you feel right now? D: I don't think I'm going to do anything right now, but to be honest, I just don't know. N: Okay, in that case I think it's important you get seen as soon as possible. In the meantime, I think it would be safer for you to wait in one of the cubicles. If you have a strong urge to leave, I'd like you to tell one of the staff. D: Okay, thanks. N: Although you've come here because of concerns about your mental health, we always take people's blood pressure, pulse and temperature, and ask a little bit about any physical health problems. Is that okay? D: Sure, no problem.

It should be emphasised that the use of good engagement skills did not require a great deal more time. The key points to note regarding the differences between A and B are:

* *The use of open questions*: In A, the nurse uses too many closed questions (Do you …? Have you …?), which elicit minimal responses from the patient. In B, more information is elicited using open questions (What …? Tell me …? How …?).

- *The use of 'why' questions*: In A, the nurse frames some of the question using 'why'. Why questions, particularly when used with the wrong tone of voice, can sound interrogative and result in the patient feeling judged.
- *The use of empathic statements or reflections*: In B, the nurse uses these skills ('It sounds really tough'. 'So, there's been a lot of difficult things happening'. 'I know this can be difficult to talk about') and thus demonstrates a sensitivity to and an understanding of David's situation.
- *Timing tasks*: In B, the nurse starts with the patient's agenda and postpones the tasks (physical observations and questions about physical health) until the end. In A, the nurse switches between asking about the reasons for presenting and task, which might appear dismissive.
- *Risk management*: In A, the nurse does not elicit from David the doubts he has about his immediate safety. In B, this is achieved by the nurse responding to a verbal cue ('I suppose I should'. 'You sound a bit reluctant'). As a result, David is placed in a safer environment while awaiting a specialist assessment. This highlights the importance of active listening and having open conversations about suicide and immediate risk. Some clinicians worry that this will increase the likelihood of the person acting on suicidal thoughts, however, the opposite is the case, in that open conversations not only help the patient feel more contained but also help facilitate the appropriate level of care required (Dazzi *et al.*, 2014).

Talking with a person experiencing acute psychosis

Case study 2.4   Carl

Carl is a 22-year-old university student who has been brought to the ED by the police. They found him wandering near the docks, appearing frightened and distracted. The police are unable to stay with Carl in the ED. After they leave, Carl's behaviour becomes more disturbed. He is increasingly suspicious, alluding to a bizarre-sounding plot against him. He also appears to be responding to voices. A doctor approaches him about taking bloods and doing an ECG, however, he becomes agitated stating that: 'You want to kill me.'

The term 'psychosis' broadly refers to a loss of contact with reality (NICE, 2014). In Carl's case, this includes conspiratorial beliefs that may be delusional and auditory hallucinations. Delusions and auditory hallucinations are both symptoms of schizophrenia, however, they can also be features of transient conditions, for example, delirium and drug-induced psychosis. Engagement with Carl to develop trust will be crucial in his care. Trust is particularly important here because he is frightened about talking to people conspiring against him and being harmed.

Compare the two ways in which the doctor engages with Carl (Table 2.2).

Table 2.2 Poor and good engagement with Carl

A Poor engagement	B Good engagement
C: The problem is nobody believes me when I say this stuff. The voices are real, they want to kill me. Dr: How can that be true? C: Because I hear them saying it all the time. Dr: Don't you think it's more likely that you're unwell at the moment? That's why you're in hospital. C: What do you mean unwell? I'm not unwell. You don't believe me either. Dr: Well, the main thing now is to get these tests done. C: No way. Dr: It's really important, come on let's get this done. C: I said no way. You're all part of this. Dr: We're really not. We're just doing our job. C: Yeah, right, well, maybe you work for them. I'm not staying here a minute longer.	C: The problem is nobody believes me when I say this stuff. The voices are real, they want to kill me. Dr: I can see how distressing this is for you. What can we do to make you less distressed? C: Just believe me when I say they're going to kill me. Dr: You sound totally convinced. C: One hundred per cent. Dr: No wonder you're so frustrated then when people don't believe you. It also sounds frightening. C: It is. Dr: You looked frightened when I talked about those tests. I just want to reassure we're not going to harm you. C: Why do you want to do tests on me? Dr: You're in hospital and we're concerned about your well-being. These tests are just a way of checking that your health is okay. C: Alright.

The key differences between these scenarios are:

- The doctor in B uses reflective statements to convey understanding and build trust.
- The doctor in B gently tests the strength of Carl's beliefs ('You sound totally convinced'), whereas the doctor in A falls into the trap of contesting the reality of Carl's beliefs ('How can that be true?' Don't you think it's more likely that you're unwell at the moment?').
- The issue of the tests is pushed by the doctor in A, justified with 'We're just doing our job' whereas the doctor in B builds good engagement before broaching the subject of the tests.

As well as increasing the likelihood of absconding, poor engagement with psychotic patients is also likely to result in agitation and behavioural disturbance.

Table 2.3 highlights some principles for supporting people with behavioural disturbance, particularly in the context of psychosis, although they have broader application.

Table 2.3 Principles for supporting people with behavioural disturbance

Do	Do not
Speak clearly in short sentences using simple language	Use jargon or stigmatising terms
Express empathy and validate how the patient feels about their experience	Collude or argue with the patient about their beliefs
Use reflection and summaries to confirm your understanding	Avoid speaking to the patient because they are difficult to understand
Remain calm, polite, and respectful	Use threatening or aggressive body language
Inform the person of what you are doing and what to expect	Assume the patient is unable to understand
Assess capacity for each decision	Assume the patient lacks capacity for all treatment decisions
Explain clinical plans, what to expect, and carry them out as explained	Cancel investigations and change plans without informing the patient
Reduce sensory overload (for example, bright lights, noises) and, if possible and safe, consider moving to a quiet space	Disrupt the patient's sleep-wake cycle
Try to understand a patient's wishes and apologise if you say something to upset the patient	Express anger or frustration to the patient if they upset you
Try to use the same staff to treat a patient so they can build rapport	Let multiple people lead a consultation or talk to a patient at one time
Pre-empt 'flashpoints' where distress may be heightened (last-minute changes to plans, staff changes, bad news, investigations) and consider how these can be best communicated or managed	Wait until behavioral disturbance occurs to engage with a patient
Build a rapport with patients early in their stay	Only engage in tasks at the expense of building rapport
Treat comorbidities, for example, pain	Ignore comorbidities

Assessment

Triage

Triage is often the first assessment in ED. For those presenting with mental health problems, some form of screening tool is often used as part of this, for example, the Risk Assessment Matrix (Patel, Harrison and Bruce-Jones, 2009), which uses a traffic light system to determine acuity. By necessity, such tools need to be highly sensitive to, and of limited specificity to, risk. This means that relatively few people will be triaged as low risk, for example, someone who has engaged in minor self-harm, has no further thought to harm themselves, who is well supported in the community, and is accompanied by a responsible adult. The majority of presentations will be referred for a specialist mental health assessment. This is similar to how people presenting with physical symptoms are treated. That is, ruling out potentially fatal diagnoses despite them being unlikely. Triage screening tools have limited value; they do not fully assess risk but can support ongoing care planning. 'High risk' individuals can be prioritised for assessment, nursed in an area with good observation, and, in some cases, have a 1:1 nurse allocated to them.

Mental health assessment as part of a medical examination

Diagnostic overshadowing

Distinguishing between organic and functional causes of 'psychiatric' symptoms is challenging. History of mental disorder can create assumptions about this being the cause of a presentation, and behavioural disturbance can lead to under-investigation, causing premature diagnostic closure and misdiagnosis. If you have a mental disorder, you are more likely to require care for, and die prematurely from physical illness, than someone with no mental disorder (Correll et al., 2017; John et al., 2018; Thornicroft, 2013). Furthermore, underlying physical health problems can present as mental disorders (for example, delirium, encephalitis) and vice versa (for example, catatonia, somatoform disorders). Evidence of fluctuation, impaired level of consciousness, cognitive impairment, and older age of onset are, for example, suggestive of organic cause, however, the absence of these features does not guarantee a functional cause.

Finding the balance between under- and over-investigation is difficult. Thorough history taking (including collateral history), examination (particularly looking for neurological signs or evidence of systemic causes), and appropriate investigation (for example, infection and metabolic screening, head imaging, lumbar puncture) can swing the balance of diagnostic probability towards or away from a functional illness. Pattern recognition is a valuable part of medical practice, however, where diagnostic uncertainty exists, unconscious biases can unduly influence management plans. It is well recognised that marginalised groups receive poorer healthcare (King's Fund, 2021), therefore, it is important to ask yourself whether you would be treating this patient the same if they had different characteristics (for example, if they were white, from a different social class, did not use drugs or did not have a history of mental illness) and ensure any differences in treatment are clearly justified. Close collaboration with other medical teams and, particularly neurology, is invaluable to appropriate management.

Case study 2.5 is typical of one in which diagnostic overshadowing might occur. Although there is a history of psychosis, Reggie's current presentation warrants further investigation. If he is deemed to lack capacity to consent to such investigations, a best interests decision will need to be made (see the section 'Capacity to consent to treatment').

Case study 2.5   Reggie

Reggie is a 60-year-old man who has had several episodes of drug-induced psychosis in the past. The last was 15 years ago. He has been brought to ED by his wife. She reports a marked change in his behaviour over the past two days with him becoming preoccupied that the neighbours are spying on him, stating he has seen 'rats and cockroaches' in their house, which he believes the neighbours put there. Reggie appears tense and distractible, pacing around the department and, at one point, shouting at another patient. His speech is fast, with normal tonal variation and varies from quiet to shouting. It is impossible to follow Reggie's train of thought; he jumps from themes of police brutality to the neighbours to one of the paramedics in the department. He is aware he is in hospital but is disorientated to time. His wife reports that he fell last week but did not seek help. He refuses investigations and shouts incoherently at the doctor who tries to perform a blood test.

History taking

Much of the history taking is like other presentations (Table 2.4), while having a psychiatric focus, for example, specifically asking about history of mental health problems when assessing past medical history, as this will not always automatically be volunteered by patients.

Additionally, there are key pieces of information one should collect to inform ongoing care, namely, the mental state examination, capacity to consent to treatment and an assessment of risk.

Mental state examination (MSE)

Documenting how the patient is presenting to you will offer insight into their current mental state (Box 2.1) and inform diagnosis, risk assessment and ongoing care. With multiple assessments by different assessors, recognition of significant fluctuations in presentation is difficult without documentation. For example, someone reporting suicidal thoughts would give greater cause for concern should they present as dishevelled, distracted, closed in posture and flat in affect, than if they were well kempt, making good eye contact, smiling occasionally and attentive. However, the histories themselves may be similar.

Table 2.4   Adaptation of standard medical history for mental health presentations

History	Details
History of presenting complaint	Self-harm/suicide (thoughts, intent, plans)/hopelessness Common symptoms: • Change in mood/energy/enjoyment levels • Sleep/appetite disturbance • Persecutory or grandiose ideas/hallucinations Precipitants to current presentation Perpetuating factors/current stressors Where relevant: circumstances of DSH/suicide attempt, including intent/planning/help seeking/current view
Past medical (and psychiatric) history	Past psychiatric history including community support/admissions Current mental health support History of self-harm Chronic or recent physical illness/pain/injury
Medication	Recent changes to prescription/doses (can precipitate delirium, Neuroleptic Malignant Syndrome (NMS), serotonin syndrome)
Family history	History of suicide increases risk
Social history	Social support/important relationships Children/carer for under-18s Employment/education Drug and alcohol use Forensic history ('ever in trouble with the police?')

Box 2.1   MSE as applied to Reggie

- *Appearance and behaviour*: No sign of self-neglect. Poor eye contact. Tense and distractible. Scowling. Verbally aggressive. Pacing around the department. Resistant to care.
- *Speech*: Normal tonal variation, pressured, marked variation in volume.
- *Mood*: Subjective: declined to answer questions. Objective: irritable. No clear evidence of affective disturbance.
- *Thought content*: Preoccupied with his neighbours spying on him and police brutality. At present, it is unclear if these are delusional. There is no evidence of suicidal ideation. His wife has expressed concerns that he might harm the neighbours.
- *Thought form*: Flight of ideas.
- *Perception*: It is unclear if he is responding to external stimuli. His reports of seeing rats and cockroaches might indicate recent visual hallucinations.
- *Cognition*: Orientated to place and person. Disorientated to time. Poor attention span.
- *Insight*: Appears to have no insight into recent changes.

Capacity to consent to treatment

A patient's capacity will influence how treatment can be provided (Figure 2.1). It will also influence where they should receive treatment and inform your response should a patient later refuse treatment or leave the department. It may be acceptable to ask a patient who has capacity to return to the waiting room while waiting for further review by the psychiatric team, whereas asking the same of someone who is unable to weigh the pros and cons of treatment may increase the risk of absconding and not be deemed to be in their best interests.

Figure 2.1 Capacity assessment

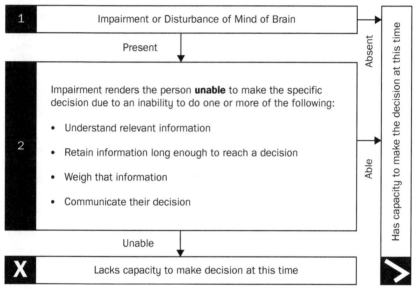

Risk assessment

The term 'risk assessment' is something of a misnomer. The ability to predict risks, for example, suicide and violence, using various screening tools and rating criteria is poor (Ryan *et al.*, 2010). However, recognising the limitations of risk assessment is an important starting point when discussing mental health assessment processes. Far more helpful than risk assessment tools is the full psychosocial assessment, which seeks to consider how the individual risk factors and stressors a person presents with can be safely mitigated against. Such assessments take time and require specialist skill and are usually carried out by the Liaison Psychiatry team or the Crisis Resolution Home Treatment team (for further discussion and exploration, see Chapter 3). Despite the limitations of risk assessment, it still has some role in guiding treatment, for example, how to respond should a patient later choose to leave the department.

When assessing risks to the patient, systematically consider the likelihood and likely severity of a risk occurring in each of the domains (Box 2.2).

Previous behaviour is the strongest predictor of future risk across domains. Mental illness, cognitive impairment and substance misuse tend to increase all risks. Good risk assessments identify factors that increase risk (for example, drug use) *and* state how these can be mitigated against (for example, support to access substance misuse services).

Box 2.2   Risk domains

- *To self*: This includes risk of DSH and suicide as well as accidental harm, for example, due to impulsivity or self-neglect related to cognitive impairment.
- *To others*: Much of the increased risk of violence to others associated with mental illness is explained by confounders, for example, alcohol or drug use, socio-economic deprivation, and victimisation (Elbogen and Johnson, 2009). However, persecutory ideas, in people with a history of violence, may increase risk (Van Dongen, Buck and Van Marle, 2012).
- *From others*: Patients may be vulnerable to exploitation from or assault by others because of their mental state, lack of capacity, cognitive impairment, or physical comorbidities. Serious mental illness increases risk of being a victim of serious crime 11-fold (Varshney *et al.*, 2016).
- *Deterioration in mental state*: Consider whether there are factors which make such a deterioration probable. For example, in a stable patient with a history of mental disorder whose medication needs to stop due to side effects, or who is prescribed medication which may precipitate relapse, such as steroids.

Assessing deliberate self-harm and suicide

Suicidal thoughts and DSH are common, with population estimates of 17 per cent and 6.4 per cent respectively (McManus *et al.*, 2019). In 2019, the suicide rate in England and Wales was 11.0 deaths per 100,000 population (Office for National Statistics, 2020). The majority of people who harm themselves or experience suicidal thoughts never come to medical attention, yet DSH accounts for over 225,000 presentations per year to ED in England alone, at a cost of over £128 million (Tsiachristas *et al.*, 2020). Suicidal thoughts and DSH can occur in the absence of a mental disorder (Hawton *et al.*, 2013), though they are more common in people experiencing anxiety disorders, affective disorders, psychosis, substance misuse and personality disorders, with repeat attendances being associated with personality and anxiety disorders (Haw *et al.*, 2001; Olfson, Marcus and Bridge, 2013). Given this, and the concern that such presentations often cause, a more detailed discussion of the assessment of DSH and suicide is warranted.

Deliberate self-harm

During assessments it is worth thinking about DSH in the broadest sense, which can include behaviours that are to some degree socially acceptable, for example, risk taking behaviours such as driving too fast, unsafe sex, and excessive use of alcohol, non-prescribed drugs, and prescribed medications (Noonan, 2013). Nevertheless, it is the more overt forms of DSH, such as cutting, burning, and insertion of foreign objects, that usually require treatment in an ED. Understanding what DSH means to the patient is an important part of the assessment.

According to an international survey (Madge *et al.*, 2008), the most common reasons for self-harm are:

1 Relief from 'a terrible state of mind' (this can include wanting to escape intense feelings of distress, frustration and being out of control, or wanting to feel emotions or ground oneself when in a state of numbness or dissociation).
2 Wanting to die.
3 As a form of self-punishment.

Although the majority of people who harm themselves do so without suicidal intent, it should be emphasised that a history of DSH is associated with an increased risk of death by suicide (Noonan, 2013). Therefore, it is important to be alert to a change in the meaning the patient attaches to DSH, for example, has it now become a rehearsal for a suicide attempt? As such, it is crucial to ask: 'What did you want to happen when you injured yourself?' Irrespective of the reason, it is essential that the patient is treated with dignity and respect. As discussed earlier, many people who attend an ED are concerned about how they will be perceived and treated. Those presenting with DSH are no exception. Indeed, many are embarrassed or ashamed by having to attend.

The medical management of DSH will be determined by the type and severity of the injury. Consent must be obtained before treatment. With respect to psychological management, National Institute for Clinical Excellence guidelines (NICE, 2004) recommend a psychosocial assessment by a mental health specialist following episodes of DSH. These options should be discussed with the patient. In the ED however, a specialist assessment may be unhelpful, for example, if the patient is a very frequent attender and there are relatively few changes in the presentations over time. In such cases, a care plan for frequent attenders can be beneficial (see case study 2.6).

Case study 2.6   Chloe

Chloe is a 24-year-old woman with a diagnosis of Emotionally Unstable Personality Disorder (EUPD). She has had over 30 attendances to the ED in the last 6 months with episodes of DSH. She usually attends during the night when she feels most lonely. If she is unable to remain in hospital overnight, she often becomes very distressed, sometimes resulting in further DSH in the ED. She is usually keen to see the liaison psychiatry team in the hope that they will admit her to a psychiatric hospital, something that her Care Coordinator refuses to do because in the past admissions have undermined her coping mechanisms, resulting in further self-harm.

Clinicians should, however, be mindful of complacency with patients like Chloe and refer for specialist assessment if there is a significant change in their presentation. For those people attending frequently who are not referred, other relevant professionals should be informed of their presentation.

Suicide

Clinicians should also be aware of the risk of suicide (case study 2.7).

Case study 2.7   Charlie

Charlie is a 49-year-old man who has been brought to the ED by ambulance because of poorly controlled diabetes. He alludes to some suicidal thoughts to the paramedics. Charlie is single, lives alone, has few friends, and has not been able to work for 5 years having been involved in an RTA, resulting in chronic pain. His father committed suicide when Charlie was 17.

At face value, there are reasons to be concerned about Charlie's risk of suicide. He has a range of actuarial risk factors. That is, factors that statistically increase the likelihood of suicide (sex, age, social isolation, unemployment, physical co-morbidity, and a family history of suicide). One of the limitations of the actuarial approach to risk assessment is that it says little about individual drivers for suicide, which are central to good risk assessment. Some theorists have refined risk assessment by focusing on a specific risk factor or cluster of factors that are purported to drive suicidal action. Beck (1986) emphasised the significance of hopelessness, the belief that one's situation cannot improve. Joiner (2005) focused on the co-existence of thwarted effectiveness (the sense that one has become a burden to others), thwarted connectedness (the sense that one does not belong), and the acquired ability to enact lethal self-injury. The latter is akin to desensitisation to pain, resulting from, for example, a history of self-harm, involvement in abusive relationships, or combat trauma.

A detailed exploration of drivers of suicidal action should be part of a specialist assessment. Although ED clinicians should take account of actuarial risk factors, an exploration of the domains in Table 2.5 provides a better foundation for an initial risk assessment.

The above factors are assessed in conjunction with the patient's history and MSE, which can form the basis of a management plan during the patient's stay in the ED. In cases where there is more immediate risk, a proactive management plan must be put in place. This should include the level of observation required, whether anxiolytic medication is necessary, and a contingency plan, should the patient wish to leave or abscond.

Table 2.5 Suicide risk assessment

Element to be assessed	Questions to ask
Ideation	Are they experiencing suicidal thoughts? How long for? Are the thoughts changing, for example, in frequency and/or intensity?
Intent	Are they thinking about acting on suicidal thoughts? How likely is it that they will? Why now?
Plan	Have they formulated a plan? Are they rehearsing the plan, for example, visiting places they could jump from? Is there a timeframe?
Means	Do they have the means to enact the plan, for example, stockpiling medication for an overdose or a rope for hanging?
Behavioural indicators	Have they been putting their affairs in order, for example, making a will or giving away possessions? If they are very agitated, is this because of overwhelming thoughts about suicide?
Protective factors	Are there aspects of their life that might mitigate the risk of suicide, for example, children, religious faith, aspirations, or goals?

Treatment refusal and the legal framework for care

Clinicians should also know what to do if a patient refuses treatment and wishes to leave (case study 2.8).

Case study 2.8 Sophia

Sophia is a 24-year-old woman who was diagnosed with EUPD last year. She was under the community mental health team at the time but was discharged after a period of non-engagement. She attends the ED after her friend called an ambulance because Sophia had cut her arm and inserted a razor under her skin. She consents to blood tests that show her paracetamol levels are very high, which could result in liver failure and death if untreated. She admits to having taken an overdose of 64 paracetamol 4 hours ago. She understands the consequences and does not want treatment for the overdose. She calmly explains that she has had suicidal thoughts for years but having recently separated from her partner, she no longer feels life is worth living and wishes to die. The notes indicate she has expressed a wish not to receive treatment for overdose at previous appointments with the mental health team.

Forcing someone who has capacity to receive care against their wishes is assault. The majority of people presenting to the ED have capacity to decide about treatment and consent to it. Those who lack capacity, for example, due to being unconscious or intoxicated can be treated under the Mental Capacity Act if this is in their best interests. However, a minority of people arrive at the ED not wanting treatment, or later withdraw their consent. In many cases, after a kind and supportive discussion, such patients independently change their mind. When this does not happen, there are legal, practical, and ethical challenges for ED clinicians. The latter is beyond the scope of this chapter but are touched upon in Chapter 6.

Legal challenges

Consideration should be given to whether there is a legal framework under which care can be given, such as the Mental Capacity Act (MCA) or the Mental Health Act (MHA),

Mental Capacity Act (MCA)

Does the patient have capacity? The responsibility for this decision sits with the person providing treatment, however, where there is a possibility of mental disorder resulting in a lack of capacity, it is valuable to seek the support of the psychiatric team and conduct a joint assessment. Assessing the presence of a disturbance of mind or brain, and a patient's ability to understand, retain and communicate a decision is relatively straightforward. However, assessing the impact of mental disorder on the ability to weigh a decision is more difficult. In Sophia's case, she is presenting as calm, gives a clear account of her weighing process, and has expressed these wishes when not distressed, which makes it challenging to argue she lacks capacity.

Mental Health Act (MHA)

The use of the MHA to treat physical presentations is very limited. It is specifically restricted to the treatment of physical symptoms that are a *direct consequence* of a mental illness. For example, refeeding after a period of dietary restriction in someone with anorexia. Treatment is not possible when symptoms are influenced by the mental disorder, for example, not taking insulin for diabetes because of a delusion of invincibility, or when a physical illness causes symptoms of mental disorder, for example, hyperthyroidism. There is, however, a legal basis for treating Sophia because:

- Sophia has a mental disorder (EUPD).
- Self-harm is a symptom of EUPD.
- The EUPD gave rise to the overdose and subsequent paracetamol toxicity for which treatment is being refused.

If, however, Sophia did not have this diagnosis, it would be more difficult to justify this causality. Furthermore, had Sophia presented only with the insertion of razor blades, it is unlikely that detention under the MHA would be considered because this could be monitored in the community. This is in keeping with the principle of providing, where possible, the least restrictive care.

Another challenge facing ED clinicians is the legal status of the patient prior to the MHA assessment taking place. Patients in the ED are *not* yet admitted to hospital, which means that Section 5(2) holding powers of the MHA cannot be used, nor can patients be detained in the ED. Furthermore, even if the patient is transferred to a ward and detained under Section 5(2), this would not cover treatment. This means clinicians must rely on the grey area of common law to temporarily restrict a patient while awaiting the MHA assessment. However, common law can only be used to protect a patient's life, or prevent significant harm to others, where the risk is considered immediate, and the response (for example, restraint) is considered proportionate to that risk. When making such decisions, seek senior input as soon as practicable (Royal College of Emergency Medicine, 2017; 2020).

The decision not to treat

When making the decision not to treat a patient who is likely to die as a result, a multi-disciplinary approach is required, involving senior colleagues. The Trust legal department should also be consulted, and they can provide assistance should the case need to go to the Court of Inherent Jurisdiction (where a patient has capacity), although both are rarely required.

Practical challenges

The main practical challenge for ED clinicians when providing treatment under a legal framework is how this can be carried out with an objecting patient. In some cases, the containment of a legal framework enables the patient to accept treatment. If not, there may be risks to the patient (because of delays in lifesaving treatment), and to other patients and staff (because of aggression/violence). The risks of delaying treatment need to be weighed against the potential psychological and physical consequences of enforcing treatment. If a delay is deemed too risky, once a legal framework is in place, sedation may be necessary to enable treatment. In extreme cases, it may be necessary to use multiple sedative drugs or even a general anaesthetic, therefore, early liaison with the anaesthetic team can be helpful. When there are risks to others, security and police involvement might be required. If the patient absconds or is allowed to leave (because it is deemed too risky to prevent this from happening), an urgent police response should be requested.

Conclusion

Given some of the challenges discussed in this chapter, some clinicians might question if the ED is an appropriate place for people in mental health crises to be seen. In response to this, it should be emphasised that there are times when it is the most appropriate place, for example, when medical treatment is required following an overdose or when investigations are required because of an acute change in a person's mental state. Moreover, as we have highlighted, physical illness and mental disorder commonly co-exist. The overlap between symptoms of mental and physical disorders in the ED contrasts with the geographical divide between many psychiatric and physical inpatient settings in the UK. For this reason, it is essential that ED clinicians develop skills to work more effectively with those patients presenting with mental disorders.

Although the ED does play a crucial role in the management of some mental health crises, it is essential that other services do not lose sight of the challenges such crises pose for patients and ED clinicians. The ED relies on other parts of the system to function well. This includes the avoidance of inappropriate signposting of people with mental health problems to ED, the prompt attendance of externally based teams when their involvement is required, and ensuring that there are sufficient psychiatric beds available to prevent those awaiting admission from inordinate delays in ED. When these and other failings occur, managing patients in mental crises in ED becomes unworkable rather than merely challenging.

Further reading

- **Quality Standards for Liaison Psychiatry Service:**
  Psychiatric Liaison Accreditation Network (PLAN): Quality Standards for Liaison Psychiatry Service. Available at: https://www.rcpsych.ac.uk/docs/default-source/improving-care/ccqi/quality-networks/psychiatric-liaison-services-plan/quality-standards-for-liaison-psychiatry-services—sixth-edition20209b6be47cb0f249f697850e1222d6b6e1.pdf?sfvrsn=1ddd53f2_0
- **Treatment pathway for urgent and emergency liaison mental health services:**
  NHS England, the National Collaborating Centre for Mental Health and NICE (2016) *Achieving Better Access to 24/7 Urgent and Emergency Mental Health Care – Part 2: Implementing the Evidence-based Treatment Pathway for Urgent and Emergency Liaison Mental Health Services.* Available at: https://www.england.nhs.uk/wpcontent/uploads/2016/11/lmhs-guidance.pdf

References

Beck, A.T. (1986) Hopelessness as a predictor of eventual suicide. *Annals of the New York Academy of Sciences*, 487(1), 90–96.
Correll, C.U., Solmi, M., Veronese, N., Bortolato, B., Rosson, S., Santonastaso, P., Thapa-Chhetri, N., Fornaro, M., Gallicchio, D., Collantoni, E., ... and Stubbs, B. (2017)

Prevalence, incidence and mortality from cardiovascular disease in patients with pooled and specific severe mental illness: A large-scale meta-analysis of 3,211,768 patients and 113,383,368 controls. *World Psychiatry*, 16(2), 163–180.

Dazzi, T., Gribble, R., Wessely, S. and Fear, N.T. (2014) Does asking about suicide and related behaviours induce suicidal ideation? What is the evidence? *Psychological Medicine*, 44(16), 3361–3363.

Elbogen, E.B. and Johnson, S.C. (2009) The intricate link between violence and mental disorder: Results from the National Epidemiologic Survey on Alcohol and Related Conditions. *Archives of General Psychiatry*, 66(2), 152–161.

Green, H. (2018) Team splitting and the 'borderline personality': A relational reframe. *Psychoanalytic Psychotherapy*, 32(3), 249–266.

Haw, C., Hawton, K., Houston, K. and Townsend, E. (2001) Psychiatric and personality disorders in deliberate self-harm patients. *British Journal of Psychiatry*, 178(1), 48–54.

Hawton, K., Saunders, K., Topiwala, A. and Haw, C. (2013) Psychiatric disorders in patients presenting to hospital following self-harm: A systematic review. *Journal of Affective Disorders*, 151(3), 821–830.

House, A. and Akagi, H. (2012) Basic skills and competencies in liaison psychiatry. In E. Guthrie, S. Rao and M. Temple (eds) *Seminars in Liaison Psychiatry*. London: The Royal College of Psychiatrists, pp. 1–14.

John, A., McGregor, J., Jones, I., Lee, S.C., Walters, J.T.R., Owen, M.J., O'Donovan, M., DelPozo-Banos, M., ... and Lloyd, K. (2018) Premature mortality among people with severe mental illness: New evidence from linked primary care data. *Schizophrenia Research*, 199, 154–162.

Joiner, T. (2005) *Why People Die by Suicide*. Cambridge, MA: Harvard University Press.

King's Fund (2021) *The Health of People from Ethnic Minority Groups in England*. Available at: https://www.kingsfund.org.uk/publications/health-people-ethnic-minority-groups-england (accessed 10 June 2021).

Koning, K.L., McNaught, A. and Tuffin, K. (2018) Emergency department staff beliefs about self-harm: A thematic framework analysis. *Community Mental Health Journal*, 54(6), 814–822.

Leigh, H. (2015) The function of consultation-liaison psychiatry. In H. Leigh and J. Streltzer (eds) *Handbook of Consultation-Liaison Psychiatry*. New York: Springer International Publishing, pp. 11–14.

Madge, N., Hewitt, A., Hawton, K., Wilde, E.J.D., Corcoran, P., Fekete, S., Heeringen, K.v., Leo, D.D. and Ystgaard, M. (2008) Deliberate self-harm within an international community sample of young people: Comparative findings from the Child and Adolescent Self-harm in Europe (CASE) Study. *Journal of Child Psychology and Psychiatry*, 49(6), 667–677.

Mental Health Act (1983) Available at: https://www.legislation.gov.uk/ukpga/1983/20/contents (accessed 8 January 2021).

McManus, S., Gunnell, D., Cooper, C., Bebbington, P.E., Howard, L.M., Brugha, T., Jenkins, R., Hassiotis, A., ... and Appleby, L. (2019) Prevalence of non-suicidal self-harm and service contact in England, 2000–14: Repeated cross-sectional surveys of the general population. *The Lancet: Psychiatry*, 6(7), 573–581.

Millard, C. (2015) *A History of Self-Harm in Britain: A Genealogy of Cutting and Overdosing*. Basingstoke: Palgrave Macmillan.

Miller, W. and Rollnick, S. (2013) *Motivational Interviewing: Helping People Change*. New York: The Guilford Press.

National Collaborating Centre for Mental Health UK (2004) Self-harm: The short-term physical and psychological management and secondary prevention of self-harm in primary and secondary care. Available at: https://www.ncbi.nlm.nih.gov/books/ NBK56385/ (accessed 2 May 2021).

NHS Digital (2020) Hospital Accident and Emergency Activity 2019–20. Available at: https://digital.nhs.uk/data-and-information/publications/statistical/hospital-accident–emergency-activity/2019-20 (accessed 2 April 2021).

NHS England, National Collaborating Centre for Mental Health and NICE (2016) Achieving better access to 24/7 urgent and emergency mental health care: Part 2: implementing the evidence-based treatment pathway for urgent and emergency liaison mental health services for adults and older adults. Available at: https://www.england.nhs.uk/publication/achieving-better-access-to-247-urgent-and-emergency-mental-health-care-part-2-implementing-the-evidence-based-treatment-pathway-for-urgent-and-emergency-liaison-mental-health-services-for/ (accessed 1 April 2021).

NICE (National Institute for Clinical Excellence) (2004) *Self-Harm in Over 8's: Short-Term Management and Prevention of Recurrence.* Available at: https://www.nice.org.uk/guidance/cg16 (accessed 20 April 2021).

NICE (National Institute for Clinical Excellence) (2014) *Psychosis and Schizophrenia in Adults: Prevention and Management.* Available at: https://www.nice.org.uk/guidance/cg178 (accessed 10 June 2021).

NICE (National Institute for Clinical Excellence) (2015) *Violence and Aggression: Short-Term Management in Mental Health and Community Settings.* Available at: https://www.nice.org.uk/guidance/NG10 (accessed 20 June 2021).

Noonan, I.P.S. (2013) Assessing and managing the risk of self-harm and suicide. In I.J. Norman and I. Ryrie (eds) *The Art and Science of Mental Health Nursing: A Textbook of Principles and Practice.* Maidenhead: Open University Press, pp. 252–273.

Office for National Statistics (2020) Suicides in England and Wales. Available at: https://www.ons.gov.uk/peoplepopulationandcommunity/birthsdeathsandmarriages/deaths/bulletins/suicidesintheunitedkingdom/2019registrations (accessed 20 May 2021).

Olfson, M., Marcus, S.C. and Bridge, J.A. (2013) Emergency Department recognition of mental disorders and short-term outcome of deliberate self-harm. *American Journal of Psychiatry*, 170(12), 1442–1450.

Patel, A.S., Harrison, A. and Bruce-Jones, W. (2009) Evaluation of the risk assessment matrix: A mental health triage tool. *Emergency Medicine Journal*, 26(1), 11–14.

Rayner, G., Blackburn, J., Edward, K., Stephenson, J. and Ousey, K. (2019) Emergency department nurse's attitudes towards patients who self-harm: A meta-analysis. *International Journal of Mental Health Nursing*, 28(1), 40–53.

RCP (Royal College of Psychiatry) (2020) *Quality Standards for Liaison Psychiatry Service*, 6th edn. Available at: https://www.rcpsych.ac.uk/docs/default-source/improving-care/ccqi/quality-networks/psychiatric-liaison-services-plan/quality-standards-for-liaison-psychiatry-services---sixth-edition-20209b6be47cb0f249f6978 50e1222d6b6e1.pdf?sfvrsn=1ddd53f2_0 (accessed 1 May 2021).

Ryan, C., Nielssen, O., Paton, M. and Large, M. (2010) Clinical decisions in psychiatry should not be based on risk assessment. *Australasian Psychiatry*, 18(5), 398–403.

The Royal College of Emergency Medicine (2017) *The Mental Capacity Act in Emergency Medicine Practice.* Available at: https://www.rcem.ac.uk//docs/RCEM%20Guidance/RCEM%20Mental%20Capacity%20Act%20in%20EM%20Practice%20-%20Feb%202017.pdf (accessed 2 June 2021).

The Royal College of Emergency Medicine (2020) The patient who absconds. Available at: https://www.rcem.ac.uk

Thornicroft, G. (2013) Premature death among people with mental illness. *British Medical Journal*, 346, 1–2.

Tsiachristas, A., Geulayov, G., Casey, D., Ness, J., Waters, K., Clements, C., Kapur, N., McDaid, D., ... and Hawton, K. (2020) Incidence and general hospital costs of self-harm across England: Estimates based on the multicentre study of self-harm. *Epidemiology and Psychiatric Sciences*, 29, 1–23.

Van Dongen, J.D.M., Buck, N.M.L. and Van Marle, H.J.C. (2012) The role of ideational distress in the relation between persecutory ideations and reactive aggression. *Criminal Behaviour and Mental Health*, 22(5), 350–359.

Varshney, M., Mahapatra, A., Krishnan, V., Gupta, R. and Deb, K.S. (2016) Violence and mental illness: What is the true story? *Journal of Epidemiology and Community Health*, 70(3), 223–225.

Walker, A., Barrett, J.R., Lee, W., West, R.M., Guthrie, E., Trigwell, P., Quirk, A., Crawford, M.J. and House, A. (2018) Organisation and delivery of liaison psychiatry services in general hospitals in England: Results of a national survey. *BMJ Open*, 8(8), 1–8.

Woollaston, K. and Hixenbaugh, P. (2008) 'Destructive Whirlwind': Nurses' perceptions of patients diagnosed with borderline personality disorder. *Journal of Psychiatric and Mental Health Nursing*, 15(9), 703–709.

3 The role of mental health services with crisis management

Rob Williams, Jordan Hodge and Kris Deering

In this chapter, the role and value of crisis resolution and home treatment teams (CRHTT) are explored. Focus will be on how interventions could be strengthened by the adoption of a consistent care model, alongside the application of recovery-orientated care. The chapter will also consider the underlying causes and definitions of 'crisis' in terms of a CRHTT and explore causal links with the stress vulnerability model. Furthermore, understanding of risk management theory will aim to be enhanced, specifically in relation to suicidality owing to being key to CRHTT work, while considering service user perspectives of safety. Finally, the importance of collaboration will be discussed, in respect of interprofessionalism and working alongside service users and significant others within the context of crisis management.

Mental health crisis provision: an overview

Over the last 25 years, CRHTT in the United Kingdom (UK) have evolved dramatically, from largely conceptual community (9 a.m.–5 p.m.) models in the early 1990s (Johnson, 2013) which focused on care in the 'least restrictive environment', into ambitious plans to provide 24/7 CRHTT coverage to every area in England by the end of 2021 (NHS, 2019a). To understand the development of CRHTT, the opening section of this chapter will contextualise how, and perhaps more importantly why, this seismic shift in mental health service provision occurred.

While several terminologies of mental health crisis provision exist, such as 'Intensive Treatment Team', 'Crisis Resolution Team' and 'Crisis Assessment Team', CRHTT tends to be the prevalent and preferred terminology (Mind, 2011; 2018; Ogaku *et al.*, 2018). However, there are significant variations in CRHTT service models. The Care Quality Commission (CQC) (CQC, 2015) concluded that despite consistent operational principles, i.e. providing both rapid and intensive support with the aim of preventing hospital admission, there were clear variations with delivery. Delivery involving help, care, and support to those experiencing a crisis were contingent on where they lived and point of entry to the service (CQC, 2015; Lloyd-Evans *et al.*, 2020). For instance, the complexities of visits in rural areas compared to those of their inner-city counterparts, with rural visits taking several hours and occurring less frequently than visits in urban areas (Mind, 2011).

Broadly, the overhaul of UK crisis provision followed the introduction of 'The NHS Plan' at the turn of the millennium. The plan highlighted key areas for investment in mental health services and identified that all catchment areas within England would offer CRHTT coverage (DH, 2000). Yet there was, and perhaps remains, a suggestion that evidence for both the establishment and efficacy of CRHTT required further detail, particularly descriptions about mental health treatment and outcomes (Hubbeling and Bertram, 2012). The introduction of the 'no health without mental health' strategy in 2012 recognised the role of public health agencies, setting out a more integrated approach, acknowledging the service user as an autonomous individual with agency, alongside acknowledging the impact of social factors on a crisis (DH, 2012). The advent of the Crisis Care Concordat (HM Government and Mind, 2014) continued to build upon multi-agency integration to be inclusive of health, social care, and criminal justice settings by identifying four key pathways:

- Access to support before crisis.
- Urgent and emergency access to crisis care.
- Quality of treatment and care when in crisis.
- Promoting recovery/preventing future crisis.

While championing responses to mental health crises, the Crisis Care Concordat also embraces interventions and preventative strategies. These have been recognised as a call for action for both national organisations (e.g. Public Health England) and representative bodies such as the Royal College of Psychiatrists (RCP). The aim is to ensure those requiring mental health support can access the appropriate services to reduce the further deterioration of their mental health (HM Government and Mind, 2014).

Though not necessarily a primary concern for practitioners, cost is a factor when deciding on future mental health provision. With large investments, a political focus may increase on mental health services (NHS, 2019a; Shaughnessy, 2015). In 2016, the 'Five-Year Forward View for Mental Health' was pivotal in securing an additional £1 billion in funding across the UK with the aim of improving accessibility as well as quality of mental healthcare. This, coupled with improved awareness of the prevalence of mental health issues, was a driver for the 'NHS Mental Health Implementation Plan', which reportedly secured a local investment fund worth at least £2.3 billion a year in real terms by 2023/24 (HM Government, 2021; NHS, 2019b).

The investment, however, pales into significance compared to the estimated cost that poor mental health carries. In England, it is estimated that poor mental health costs over £105 billion every year (DHSC, 2016). While approximately 23 per cent of NHS activity relates to mental health provision, spending on secondary mental health services appears less than half (NHS, 2016). Nevertheless, there remains robust and consistent evidence that CRHTT is a cost-effective intervention when compared with inpatient admission (Ford *et al.*, 2001; Johnson *et al.*, 2017; McCrone *et al.*, 2009; Paton *et al.*, 2016). These findings must be treated with some caution, as overall cost effectiveness can stem from regional variations, such as costs surrounding decreased hospital beds and whether more people are receiving a service (Hubbeling and Bertram, 2012).

Also of note, CRHTT have received criticism in recent years about failing to provide service users with continuity of care and more strikingly, given the focus on interprofessionalism, significant gaps remain with service integration (CQC, 2020; Werbeloff *et al.*, 2017). Accordingly, the UK Government has issued proposals for significant reforms to the Mental Health Act (MHA). In relation to this chapter, the new Mental Health White Paper aims to improve access to crisis services, including earlier support and alternatives to detention for individuals experiencing mental health crises (HM Government, 2021).

Defining crisis within CRHTT

Seminal work by Caplan (1964) proposed that crises occur when individuals encounter problems which they cannot resolve with their established coping mechanisms. The inability to resolve the problem(s) results in a heightened state of stress, apprehension, and emotional unrest. Situations exceeding established coping mechanisms are echoed by Roberts and Ottens (2005), who describe crisis as a period of psychological disequilibrium, also acknowledged by James and Gilliland (2016), identifying the 'perceived' intolerability of difficult situations. As Chapter 1 highlights, numerous definitions and ideas exist when encapsulating not only the complexity, but also the subjectivity of a mental health crisis. For instance, Vos, Roberts and Davies (2019) propose that people live in an 'age of crises' relating to wider, persistent, social upheavals that are intrinsically linked to personal interpretations. Adopting a more unequivocal definition, the Mental Health Foundation (2019) suggests 'a mental health crisis is an emergency that poses a direct and immediate threat to your physical or emotional wellbeing'. Essentially, within the backdrop of CRHTT, a mental health crisis means urgent help is required due to a perceived, unmanageable emotional or mental state, while characteristics of these are discussed below.

Despite the broadness of crisis definitions, there are some commonalities that CRHTT address. High levels of agitation are associated alongside acts which endanger the person or others, suicidal impulses and an overwhelming need to self-harm can be involved, as well as fear resulting from fluctuations in mental health symptoms, such as psychosis (Mind, 2011; Rethink, 2020). Crisis can also relate to wider psychosocial factors such as bereavement, financial issues, and poor housing alongside relationship difficulties (e.g. physical or emotional abuse) (WHO, 2019). The impact of the Covid-19 pandemic, for instance, has seen an additional 2.2 million adults seeking support for mental health-related difficulties since April 2020, resulting in an 8 per cent increase in treatment sessions and a record increase of 159,347 referrals to CRHTT (Royal College of Psychiatrists, 2021). While the reasons for this are diverse, increases are linked to social disconnection and isolation (Byrne, Barber and Lim, 2021), hence demonstrating the effect of social issues on a mental health crisis.

CRHTT response – is it an emergency?

At times of mental distress, the terms crisis and emergency can be indistinguishable (Brennaman, 2012). Guidance provided by the NHS often directs individuals straight to emergency departments (ED), particularly if there is a perceived risk to life (NHS, 2020). Although, as other chapters suggest, an inherent subjectivity exists with both terminologies depending on the professional service. Added complexity surrounds the perception of the service user and significant others, particularly their experiences of crisis care, and disparity between expectations of service providers and those accessing services (Brennan *et al.*, 2016). Nevertheless, there appear to be some differences between terminologies, as suggested below.

- *mental health emergency*: a life-threatening situation – an individual is threatening harm to themselves or others.
- *mental health crisis*: involves non-life-threatening situations – an individual may be presenting with extreme emotional disturbance or distress.

(Mental Health Foundation, 2019)

Interestingly, the terminology 'mental health emergency' appears almost absent in England's NHS crisis documentation (NHS, 2016; 2019a). Instead, the term 'emergency' is generally reserved for the responses required from services, rather than the presenting problem (HM Government and Mind, 2014; NHS, 2019b). According to Jones (2020), such ambiguity, coupled with the absence of agreed criteria for crisis, shifts responses towards the assessment and management of risk. While risk assessment is somewhat central to crisis intervention, there are conflicting views if it has an impact on adverse events, such as suicide (Hung *et al.*, 2012). Mulder, Newton-Howes and Coid (2018) propose that the risk factors used to predict suicide are a 'myth', often incorrectly attributing suicide due to a lack of a comprehensively written risk assessment. An over-emphasis can be placed on predictability of the assessment providing a false sense of security to CRHTT clinicians and service managers, rather than perhaps considering the benefits of the therapeutic engagement with the service user (Chan *et al.*, 2016).

The points raised are significant. CRHTT can have higher risk thresholds than other agencies which fluctuate depending on hospital bed availability, workload, and caseload management (Lombardo *et al.*, 2019) and can be a source of interprofessional conflict, especially when the role of the CRHTT is not clearly defined, resulting in inadequate interprofessional responses to service user needs (Johnson, 2013). Alternatively, CRHTT services benefit from mitigating conflict, sharing their expertise even with inappropriate referrals, offering guidance and support to partner agencies, as this can aid the service user. In short, available evidence suggests that a mental health crisis does constitute an emergency, in terms of the response required and potential risk outcomes. Nevertheless, response times fall short of those within other emergency services such as police or ambulance, with the standard CRHTT response time usually occurring 'within 2–4 hours' (NHS, 2019a; 2019b). While reasons are varied, responses can be influenced by resourcing, opaque service definition, and ongoing debate as to what constitutes a mental health crisis (Brennan *et al.*, 2016).

The purpose and value of CRHTT

CRHTT provide rapid responses to individuals experiencing episodes of mental health crisis, preferably as home treatment, without which a hospital admission may result (RCP, 2019). Home treatment holds the view that in a personal recognisable space, people are more able to flourish, especially with the support of significant others, lessening the impact of the crisis (Mind, 2018). Interventions commence with ascertaining the cause(s), including assessing psychosocial triggers, i.e. stress vulnerabilities (discussed later), and the immediacy of risks to self and others, such as suicide and violence. Interventions also involve supporting service users to develop and implement effective coping strategies, aiming to empower people, with the goal of stabilising the crisis and reducing relapse (Morant *et al.*, 2017; NICE, 2011). Responding to mental health crises can be complex and involves a unique set of actions from a multi-disciplinary team (MDT) designed to support an individual. Primarily, the decision to use a CRHTT can be broken down into two separate categories (RCP, 2016):

- containment and management of risk;
- the ability to provide therapeutic interventions.

As set out in the four principles of the Nursing and Midwifery Code (NMC, 2018), services must do all they can to support a service user and prevent the individual from experiencing or causing further harm. CRHTT are seen as the last 'least restrictive option' or 'ward in the community', in which the team have abilities, through a wide range of resources not commissioned for other services, to intensively support service users.

Containment and management of risk within CRHTT relate to mitigating behaviours that can result from mental health difficulties. These can be far-reaching, like self-harm and self-neglect, in which the CRHTT predominantly look to manage acute distress, minimise possible imminent harms, improve functioning, alongside providing an alternative to hospital admission, and problem-solve acute social and interpersonal conflicts (Tees, Esk and Wear Valleys NHS Foundation Trust, 2021). The ability to respond to these behaviours requires a reactive and often intensive set of interventions. As documented in the 'Home Treatment Accreditation Scheme', which sets out a comprehensive framework to develop CRHTT, there is a need for experienced healthcare professionals led by a consultant psychiatrist to conduct regular visits to service users (RCP, 2019). The latter is to provide care while CRHTT ideally have exclusive use of 'crisis houses' where patients can stay to convalesce from mental distress (RCP, 2019).

Providing therapeutic interventions can be contentious and difficult to achieve. For example, CRHTT requesting a Mental Health Act assessment (MHA 1983; amended 2007) can pose difficult questions about trust, engagement, and fear for the service user (Akther et al., 2019). CRHTT therapeutic interventions do not differ greatly from other mental health teams. However, the ability to intensively provide and assist with acute distress allows a rapid response, otherwise not offered by other mental health services in the community (RCP, 2019). Notably, service users, care-coordinated by clinicians from community mental health teams (CMHT), may receive bi-weekly visits. If mental health deteriorates, CRHTT intervention might be required, rapidly increasing visits up to four times per day depending on need (Chunduri et al., 2019). Interventions provided by other mental health teams might remain, but the frequency of these will increase led by the needs at the time to support the individual, to lessen further deterioration and, when possible, avoid hospital admission.

It is important to note that risk behaviours may not be the only precursor to CRHTT involvement. With current mental health funding and resource gaps, including under-recruitment (Liu et al., 2018), appropriate and designated resources could be unavailable in which support is normally provided from the referrer. This can lead to conflicts about appropriate referrals, as the CRHTT may have concerns about disrupting the continuity of care, which can, in some cases, further the mental health crisis experienced by the service user (Mahomed, 2020).

The function of the CRHTT

CRHTT services are dynamic and complex in nature, especially from those looking to make a referral or wanting to access their care. However, essentially, the intent is to offer a full holistic and interprofessional approach to crisis care (RCP, 2016). Often, CRHTT are classed as multi-disciplinary teams providing specialist care by trained practitioners in a variety of fields. Registered mental health nurses (MHN) make up most of these teams due to the medical input service users require during the crisis period (Lloyd-Evans et al., 2018). This can be via the management and reconciliation of medications. However, ensuring that a mixed bio-social and recovery model is followed, allied healthcare professionals play a pivotal role in providing care that meets the

whole needs of the individual (Bellier-Teichmann *et al.*, 2016). These can con-
sist of occupational therapists, social workers, psychological practitioners and
support workers. Ensuring that shared decision making and not a 'top-down
approach' is followed allows the review of the individual from each perspective
and discipline, as a crisis can be multifactorial (Bhugra *et al.*, 2011).

CRHTT play a significant role in supporting people with medication management. Service users in NHS mental health settings are frequently prescribed
relevant medication, such as anti-depressants, anti-psychotics, benzodiaze-
pines (sedatives) and hypnotics (to aid sleep). Medications can be administered
and managed in other secondary care services, such as CMHT, as well as in
general practice. The difference within CRHTT is the focus of acute management of psychiatric medication and the dosage range prescribed to stabilise a
crisis (Onyett *et al.*, 2008). As highlighted by NICE (2017) guidance on medication management, monitoring arrangements for restarting and initiating medications are essential. This is especially pertinent in crisis situations where
agreement to take medication can be compromised by mental distress (Sreenath
et al., 2010). Multiple visits a day, with proactive and timely medication reviews
alongside intensive monitoring of side effects, can contribute to a reduction in
severe mental health symptoms. As such, medication makes an important contribution in lessening the crisis that patients are experiencing (Murphy *et al.*,
2015).

Interprofessional working extends beyond the multidisciplinary composi-
tion of CRHTT. One of the main functions of the crisis service is to liaise and
'connect' services together to ensure that the patient is continuing to receive
care from previous or current providers such as social services and general
practice (Bridgett and Polak, 2003). Liaison and networking are crucial to meet
the needs of the individual, not merely delivered by the CRHTT, but from as
many providers as necessary, and appropriate to the needs of service users.

As noted, medication reconciliation is a major factor in successful treatment
demonstrating the importance of partnership working with other services
involved in the patient's care, such as the General Practitioner (GP). Such collaboration commences care and continues throughout to when the service user
is 'stepped down' once the crisis has stabilised. In terms of GPs, collaboration is
key, due in part to their sustained involvement that can occur throughout the
person's life. Hence a constant point of contact for health-related issues, especially involving relapse prevention and long-term recovery, as over 90 per cent
of people with mental health issues are cared for in primary care (Royal College of General Practitioners, 2017). Close support and liaison with family and
carers are also important. Often described as the 'triangle of care' in policy,
collaborating with significant others is essential for community treatment to
continue effectively and safely (Bradley, 2015). One of the drivers behind this
collaboration is the capacity of the CRHTT to offer 24-hour care, in which the
service relies on family and carers to 'bridge the gap' and provide feedback and
support, particularly when CRHTT services encounter hurdles, for example,
system pressures and capacity that impact on providing care (Bridgett and
Polak, 2003).

Stress vulnerability and CRHTT care

The stress vulnerability model proposed by Zubin and Spring (1977) has made an important contribution to understanding the antecedents of psychological and psychiatric conditions. Goh and Agius (2010) identified stress as a significant component of the aetiology of mental illnesses seen in CRHTT, notably schizophrenia, bipolar disorder, post-traumatic stress disorder (PTSD) and depression. Similarly, stress-psychopathology models suggest stress has a causal influence on the development of psychopathology (Olino, Mennies and Wojcieszak, 2020). Given that CRHTT operate within high stress situations, it is theorised that some risks like suicide are perpetuated by psychosocial adversities, suggesting a relationship with increased stress and mental health crises (van Heeringen, 2012). These potential stress factors are listed in Figure 3.1, to aid understanding of what might lead to a mental health crisis encountered by a CRHTT.

Figure 3.1 Causal factors of stress can be broken down into five distinct categories

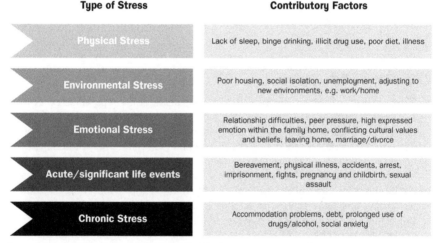

Type of Stress	Contributory Factors
Physical Stress	Lack of sleep, binge drinking, illicit drug use, poor diet, illness
Environmental Stress	Poor housing, social isolation, unemployment, adjusting to new environments, e.g. work/home
Emotional Stress	Relationship difficulties, peer pressure, high expressed emotion within the family home, conflicting cultural values and beliefs, leaving home, marriage/divorce
Acute/significant life events	Bereavement, physical illness, accidents, arrest, imprisonment, fights, pregnancy and childbirth, sexual assault
Chronic Stress	Accommodation problems, debt, prolonged use of drugs/alcohol, social anxiety

Source: Adapted from Mind (2017), NHS (2019c), Mental Health Foundation (2021).

Much discussion exists within the wider literature around perceived causes of stress, acknowledging a correlation between adaptability and coping strategies of the individual, alongside the perceived level of stress attributed to current circumstances (American Psychological Association, 2020; NHS, 2019c; Vrshek-Schallhorn et al., 2015). However, a question remains; is stress a mental health difficulty? Stress is a normal part of everyday living and can even be positive. In terms of eustress, stress can be beneficial, providing a person with excitement to engage in activities, and may help to build tolerance to adverse events (Seery, Holman and Silver, 2010). However, problems arise with the cumulative effects of stress increasing vulnerability to mental health crises (NHS, 2019c).

Approaches drawn from the stress vulnerability model have been instrumental to the development of psychosocial intervention tools, notably the 'stress bucket'; a metaphor to consider how stress can build up and be managed. The clinician asks the service user to visualise a bucket with a tap at the bottom and the bucket gradually fills up through experiences of different stressors. The service user then considers mechanisms which relieve stress, i.e. opening the tap to drain the bucket. Originally designed to explain the likelihood of developing psychotic symptoms, its application has expanded for people in crisis to understand the influences of societal and interpersonal factors on current difficulties (Brabban and Turkington, 2002; University of Bristol, 2020). Transactional models of stress and coping also place emphasis on the assessment of needs and review when considering stress causes, and these can be essential when formulating clinical responses (Liu *et al.*, 2019). Hence, understanding the subjectivity of stress responses and helping patients to develop effective coping mechanisms are pivotal to CRHTT provision (NICE, 2011; RCP, 2019). As case study 3.1 shows, it might not necessarily alleviate clinical concerns about risk, but it can help to bring about a clearer picture of what is happening for the service user.

Case study 3.1   Peter

Peter is seen following a serious attempt of suicide. It is established Peter is a 23-year-old male who has recently broke up with his partner John. Peter answers questions with mostly 'I don't know'. With concern about suicide, the clinician asks about Peter's abilities to keep himself safe. This too results in unclear responses, raising clinical fears. The clinician changes tack and explores the impact of stress. The conversation starts with Peter's views about the stress involved when intimate relationships end. Peter states everything has been more stressful since his partner left him. The clinician takes time to unpick what everything might involve and adopting the stress bucket, explores the ripple effect of the breakdown of the relationship, identifying with Peter problems at work and breakdown of friendships shared with John. While the risk of suicide remained, a clearer picture emerged through exploring stress of the impact of the relationship breakdown. In addition, rather than only assessing in terms of mental illness, exploration moved to what Peter found meaningful, to help gain more clarity about his interpretations of the crisis.

CRHTT good practice

When considering the diverse crisis definitions, alongside variations in CRHTT implementation, it becomes apparent that there is a need for a structured model of crisis intervention. While operational principles exist, i.e.

Figure 3.2 The Seven-Stage Crisis Intervention Model

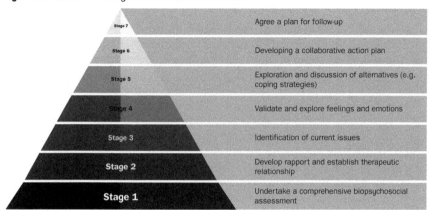

Stage 7 — Agree a plan for follow-up

Stage 6 — Developing a collaborative action plan

Stage 5 — Exploration and discussion of alternatives (e.g. coping strategies)

Stage 4 — Validate and explore feelings and emotions

Stage 3 — Identification of current issues

Stage 2 — Develop rapport and establish therapeutic relationship

Stage 1 — Undertake a comprehensive biopsychosocial assessment

Source: Adapted from Roberts and Ottens (2005, p. 7).

rapid assessment, gatekeeping/lessening hospital admissions and multidisciplinary approaches, CRHTT tend to employ broad frameworks. These are to accommodate diverse theoretical approaches with crisis management (Johnson, 2013). One such theoretical framework is the 'Seven-Stage Crisis Intervention Model', proposed by Roberts and Ottens (2005). As the title suggests, the framework shown in Figure 3.2 identifies the seven stages of interventions key to stabilising a crisis.

Roberts and Ottens (2005) recommend the priority for any crisis intervention should be a thorough assessment, considering lethality, alongside establishing whether any life-threatening actions have occurred or are imminent, e.g. self-poisoning. As such, the assessment overlaps with service users in ED and mental health liaison services (see Chapter 2). With most mental health interventions, the early establishment of a therapeutic rapport (or alliance) is key for CRHTT. Crisis interventions undertaken when there is a perceived or established therapeutic rapport between clinicians and service users appear to be effective (Farrelly *et al.*, 2015). Furthermore, CRHTT clinicians should endeavour to promote multi-agency working to maintain the therapeutic relationships that already exist between the service user and other services, especially as these services may continue to support the individual following the crisis phase, such as CMHT (HM Government and Mind, 2014; Johnson, 2013). Adherence to multi-agency working requires CRHTT clinicians to be both skilled in risk management and comfortable with positive risk-taking (Just, Palmier-Claus and Tai, 2021). That is, a multi-agency approach to taking calculated risks, such as building social networks, to ensure there is full support, whenever possible, to aid life satisfaction for the patient.

Risk management is a pivotal part of CRHTT crisis interventions, given that many patients referred experience suicidal ideation (RCP, 2019). There appears a held belief from those engaging with individuals experiencing suicidal ideation that '*most ... do not wish to die but simply cannot imagine continuing to live in their current state of psychological turmoil*' (Granello, 2010, p. 219). Furthermore, to complete suicide, an individual must not only have the desire but also overcome fears about their own death (Ma *et al.*, 2016). It is worth revisiting the work of Joiner (2005, see Chapter 2) who explored fears about death with the 'interpersonal theory of suicide'. The theory explains why individuals engage in suicidal behaviours and comprises three core components: (1) thwarted belongingness; (2) perceived burdensomeness; and (3) acquired capability (i.e. the ability to act upon suicidal ideation), a particular concern when thwarted belongingness and perceived burdensomeness co-exist. CRHTT, by their very nature, operate within the parameters of this theory (RCP, 2019). By promoting a sense of social connectedness through collaboration, not only can interventions be improved, but also undesirable outcomes, like suicide, can potentially be averted.

There is increasing debate about assimilating recovery-orientated care with risk management to cultivate collaboration (Deering *et al.*, 2019; Tickle, Brown and Hayward, 2014). While previously discussed, it is also worth revisiting recovery owing to its relevance to CRHTT care. Despite its roots in survivor movements characterised by advocacy initiatives for marginalised patients, the recovery paradigm uses a variety of personal and clinical approaches (Deegan, 1988; Slade, 2009). Clinicians attempt to draw upon service users' views with the aim of establishing what would make life more satisfying for them, alongside care using clinical expertise (Oates, Drey and Jones, 2017). Ultimately, recovery is a process, moving towards life satisfaction defined by the individual and arises irrespective of continuing mental health difficulties (Slade and Longden, 2015). Mental illness should not discourage individuals from engaging in activities that enrich their quality of life, as such, CRHTT implementing a recovery-focused approach may alleviate risks (Morrissey, Doyle and Higgins, 2018; Perkins and Repper, 2016). When given an active voice about care, i.e., in decision making and care planning, an internal shift can occur from a sense of hopelessness towards one of hope, enabling the service user to realise their potential to have a more meaningful life (Bird *et al.*, 2014; McKenna *et al.*, 2014).

Naturally, a challenge for CRHTT (as well as other mental health services) is that the recovery approach is not a panacea, nor is it without its critics. There is often an underlying assumption that mental illnesses are solvable solely through care practices, without necessarily addressing the wider societal issues which underpin them (Deering, 2016; Newman-Taylor, Maguire and Bowen, 2019; Recovery in the Bin, 2019). Even so, for recovery to flourish, people need to feel safe with risk management and crisis interventions. As described by the hierarchy of human needs, a conceptual psychological model conceived by Maslow (1954), human behaviours are ultimately determined by our desire to satisfy our needs. These 'needs' are structured in the form of a pyramid, presented in Figure 3.3.

Figure 3.3 Maslow's hierarchy of needs

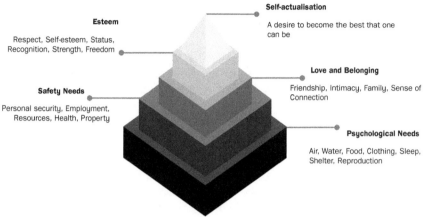

Adapted from Maslow (1954).

The relevance of the hierarchy permeates many aspects of mental health provision to this day, including the NHS Constitution as well as parallels with the recovery paradigm (DHSC, 2021; Henwood *et al.*, 2015). The most significant element of Maslow's hierarchy to CRHTT is safety. Indeed, a perceived lack of safety is one of the key contributory factors to crisis presentations (Berzins *et al.*, 2018). Safety can move beyond mitigating risk and include patients feeling safe to discuss meanings attributable to crises, and ways to engage in risk-taking to promote a satisfying life, alongside tackling issues like stress vulnerabilities, rather than limiting care to treating illness (Crowe and Deane, 2018). Moreover, recovery linked to social connectedness may alleviate alienation and strengthen the desire to live (Joiner *et al.*, 2012). Thus, building interpersonal relations, whereby individuals believe clinicians genuinely wish to help, and see themselves worthy of care, is pivotal to crisis management (Sayer, 2017). This is significant, as considering feeling oneself a burden to others increases disengagement and risk of suicide (Joiner *et al.*, 2012). However, clinical fears about blame should an adverse incident occur, and concern about patient risk illiteracies mean their views are not always obtained (Felton, Repper and Avis, 2018). Hence, it remains to be seen how the 'apparent contradictions [between risk management and recovery] can be reconciled and an approach developed which will effectively and safely support people in their recovery' (Boardman and Roberts, 2014).

In light of the fact that safety can be multifaceted whereby service users and their significant others may have different views from clinical concerns about risk, the case study of Peter is revisited below. This is to show that Peter might have seen safety in terms of psychological well-being and how the relationship breakdown generated a sense that life felt less safe.

Case study 3.2   Peter

On a home visit, covering the walls were pictures of Peter and John and it was a surprise these had not been removed. The clinician asks about the pictures, but does so tentatively as to be respectful: 'I notice there are lots of pictures on the ...'; Peter interjects, 'Stupid, right? Just a reminder ...'. 'May I ask, a reminder about what?' queries the clinician. Peter thinks about this and responds, 'A time when life made sense, when I knew what was what, I knew who I was ... now there is nothing.' 'Nothing?' asks the clinician. 'Yeah, ... nothing ... nothing is certain ...'. The clinician ponders: 'Like unstable?' 'Unstable?' questions Peter. 'I wonder if life feels unstable?' asks the clinician. Peter agrees, 'Yeah, I don't know what is what ... unstable, yeah, ... without John, life is not stable ...'. 'I guess we all have need for security ... sometimes,' raises the clinician. 'Yeah,' responds Peter. 'I wonder, Peter, what does security look like to you, any feelings maybe ...?' 'Yeah, it's about feeling safe, innit? Not feeling scared all the bloody time.'

Collaboration with family and carers

Collaboration with other services, as highlighted, is an important factor in supporting people experiencing crisis (NHS, 2019a; RCP, 2019). However, collaboration, in terms of patient-centred care, requires an ability to engage family and carers to support the process of crisis recovery. An independent inquiry, commissioned by Mind (2011), highlights the importance of family and carer connections, the trauma when such connections are severed, and increasing care provision to the person's support networks (Mind, 2011). As a main function of CRHTT, the involvement of family and carers from the outset is an integral part of community support, as it is recognised that CRHTT cannot provide full 24-hour care like hospital settings (Morant et al., 2017; NHS, 2019a; 2019b). However, whenever possible, CRHTT need to consider their service as an outlet to provide guidance and support to family and carers either over the phone, in person or through liaising with support agencies (e.g. Rethink and Mind). This is important, given significant others predominantly care for people experiencing crisis (Rethink, 2021).

Building upon the triangle of care to improve carer involvement, CRHTT should aspire to engage and develop strategies, such as guidance from the Princess Royal Trust for Carers (Carers UK, 2021). The guidance focuses on a holistic management of service user care where family and carers are at the heart of the shared decision-making process. Involvement is one of the core themes which arises from stakeholder engagement, especially involving CRHTT (Morant et al., 2017). Acute distress can impact on abilities to provide consent for significant others to be involved in care, hindering collaboration. However, rather than a foregone conclusion when first asked, consent to involve others must be reviewed, for the benefits of such collaboration can become more understood as the crisis diminishes (Rudd et al., 2009).

Brennan et al. (2016) described the experience of a family member during a crisis, noting it was '... scary, challenging, traumatic, and stressful. They associated it with feelings of anxiety, concern and hopelessness' (p. 454). Thus, understanding the physical and mental implications of caring for someone in crisis is critical, while support for family members and carers should be an operational priority for CRHTT (RCP, 2019). As highlighted in Maslow's (1954) hierarchy of needs, friendship, family and a sense of connection are important to work towards self-esteem and self-actualisation. From a CRHTT perspective, such care commences with meaningful conversations about the impact of the crisis, alongside exploring care mechanisms in place or needed, for both service users and their support networks.

Conclusion

CRHTT coverage and provision in the UK have improved greatly since their inception in the early 1990s. There is now some consistency in terms of operational principles as well as recognition from the government that avoiding hospital admission, wherever possible, is a cost-effective strategy by providing intensive support to those experiencing crisis. Nevertheless, significant shortfalls still exist in terms of the consistency of treatment models and measurable outcomes across CRHTT.

Questions remain about the CRHTT focus on risk management – particularly the predictability of risk assessments – despite a diminutive evidence base. Incorporating a recovery-focused approach to risk management, accompanied with a consistently implemented intervention framework like the Seven-Stage Crisis Intervention Model, appears a suitable step to improve the efficacy of CRHTT interventions and service user satisfaction. However, these approaches will require further research, particularly to understand more fully the integration of recovery with risk and crisis management.

The NHS Long-Term Plan (2019a) has allocated approximately £200 million of funding, with the view of transforming both urgent and emergency mental healthcare provision by 2022. Currently, proposals suggest the introduction of 'safe havens' and 'crisis cafés' across the country to provide safe spaces where people can go when in crisis, as an alternative to ED. This is a significant way forward considering the importance of social connectedness and lessening risks, notable with suicide. Such reforms will ideally form an integral component of CRHTT interventions as the UK emerges from the global pandemic. However, only time will tell the true extent of the national mental health crisis that appears to be on the horizon.

Further reading

- **Collaboration and suicide prevention:**
  Jobes, D.A. (2016) *Managing Suicidal Risk: A Collaborative Approach*, 2nd edn. New York: Guilford Press.
- **Comprehensive guide to crisis management:**

Yeager, K. and Roberts. A. (2015) *Crisis Intervention Handbook: Assessment, Treatment, and Research*, 4th edn. Oxford. Oxford University Press.
• **Overview of CRHTT:**
Johnson, S. (2008) *Crisis Resolution and Home Treatment in Mental Health*. Cambridge: Cambridge University Press.
• **The interpersonal model of suicide:**
Joiner, T. (2007) *Why People Die by Suicide*. Cambridge, MA: Harvard University Press.

References

Akther, S.F., Molyneaux, E., Stuart, R., Johnson, S., Simpson, A. and Oram, S. (2019) Patients' experiences of assessment and detention under mental health legislation: Systematic review and qualitative meta-synthesis. *British Journal of Psychiatry Open*, 5(3), 1–10.

American Psychological Association (2020) Stress in America: A national mental health crisis. APA Press release. Available at: https://www.apa.org/news/press/releases/stress/2020/report-october (accessed 1 May 2021).

Bellier-Teichmann, T., Golay, P., Bonsack, C. and Pomini, V. (2016) Patients' needs for care in public mental health: Unity and diversity of self-assessed needs for care. *Frontiers in Public Health*, 4(22), 1–8.

Berzins, K., Baker, J., Brown, M. and Lawton, R. (2018) A cross-sectional survey of mental health service users', carers' and professionals' priorities for patient safety in the United Kingdom. *Health Expectations*, 21(6), 1085–1094.

Bhugra, D., Easter, A., Mallaris, Y. and Gupta, S. (2011) Clinical decision making in psychiatry by psychiatrists. *Acta Psychiatrica Scandinavica*, 124(5), 403–411.

Bird, V., Leamy, M., Tew, J., Le Boutillier, C., Williams, J. and Slade, M. (2014) Fit for purpose? Validation of a conceptual framework for personal recovery with current mental health consumers. *The Australian and New Zealand Journal of Psychiatry*, 48(7), 644–653.

Boardman, J. and Roberts, G. (2014) *Risk, Safety and Recovery*. Available at: https://www.centreformentalhealth.org.uk/sites/default/files/2018-09/risksafetyrecovery.pdf (accessed 4 April 2021).

Brabban, A. and Turkington, D. (2002) The search for meaning: Detecting congruence between life events, underlying schema and psychotic symptoms: Formulation-driven and schema-focused cognitive behavioural therapy for a neuroleptic-resistant schizophrenic patient with a delusional memory. In A.P. Morrison (ed.) *Casebook of Cognitive Therapy for Psychosis*. New York: Brunner-Routledge, pp. 59–75.

Bradley, E. (2015) Carers and co-production: Enabling expertise through experience. *Mental Health Review Journal*, 20(4), 232–241.

Brennaman, L. (2012) Crisis emergencies for individuals with severe, persistent mental illnesses: A situation-specific theory. *Archives of Psychiatric Nursing*, 26(4), 251–260.

Brennan, A., Warren, N., Peterson, V., Hollander, Y., Boscarato, K. and Lee, S. (2016) Collaboration in crisis: Carer perspectives on police and mental health professionals' responses to mental health crises. *International Journal of Mental Health Nursing*, 25(5), 452–461.

Bridgett, C. and Polak, P. (2003) Social systems intervention and crisis resolution: Part 2 – Intervention. *Advances in Psychiatric Treatment*, 9(6), 432–438.

Byrne, A., Barber, R. and Lim, C.H. (2021) Impact of the COVID-19 pandemic: A mental health service perspective. *Progress in Neurology and Psychiatry*, 25(2), 27–33.

Caplan, G. (1964) *Principles of Preventive Psychiatry*. New York: Basic Books.

Carers UK (2021) Guidance: Princess Royal Trust for Carers. Available from: https://www.carersuk.org/ (accessed 8 May 2021).

Chan, M.K.Y., Bhatti, H., Meader, N., Stockton, S., Evans, J., O'Connor, R.C., Kapur, N. and Kendall, T. (2016) Predicting suicide following self-harm: Systematic review of risk factors and risk scales. *British Journal of Psychiatry*, 209, 277–283.

Chunduri, S., Browne, S., Pollio, D.E., Hong, B.A., Roy, W., Roaten, K., Khan, F. and North, C.S. (2019) Suicide risk assessment and management in the psychiatry emergency service: Psychiatric provider experience and perceptions. *Archives of Suicide Research*, 23(1), 1–14.

CQC (Care Quality Commission) (2015) Right here, right now: People's experiences of help, care and support during a mental health crisis. Available at: https://www.cqc.org.uk/sites/default/files/20150611_righthere_mhcrisiscare_summary_3.pdf (accessed 23 May 2021).

CQC (Care Quality Commission) (2020) *State of Care: Annual Assessment of Health and Social Care in England*. Available at: https://www.cqc.org.uk/publications/major-report/state-care (accessed 1 May 2021).

Crowe, S. and Deane, F. (2018) Characteristics of mental health recovery model implementation and managers' and clinicians' risk aversion. *The Journal of Mental Health Training, Education and Practice*, 13(1), 22–33.

Deegan, P.E. (1988) Recovery: The lived experience of rehabilitation. *Psychosocial Rehabilitation Journal*, 11(4), 11–19.

Deering, K. (2016) Neoliberalism and self-management: The case for social justice. *Mental Health Nursing Journal*, 36(4), 10–12.

Deering, K., Pawson, C., Summers, N. and Williams, J. (2019) Patient perspectives of helpful risk management practices within mental health services: A mixed studies systematic review of primary research. *Journal of Psychiatric and Mental Health Nursing*, 26(5–6), 185–197.

Department of Health (2000) *The NHS Plan: A Plan for Investment, a Plan for Reform*. Available at: https://webarchive.nationalarchives.gov.uk/20130124064356/http://www.dh.gov.uk/prod_consum_dh/groups/dh_digitalassets/@dh/@en/@ps/documents/digitalasset/dh_118522.pdf (accessed 23 April 2021).

Department of Health (2012) No health without mental health: Implementation framework. Available at: https://www.gov.uk/government/publications/mental-health-implementation-framework (accessed 25 April 2021).

Department of Health and Social Care (2016) New investment in mental health services. Available at: https://www.gov.uk/government/news/new-investment-in-mental-health-services (accessed 11 June 2021).

Department of Health and Social Care (2021) *The NHS Constitution for England*. HM Government. DHSC. Available at: https://www.gov.uk/government/publications/the-nhs-constitution-for-england/the-nhs-constitution-for-england (accessed 25 April 2021).

Farrelly, S., Lester, H., Rose, D., Birchwood, M., Marshall, M., Waheed, W., Henderson, R. C., … and Thornicroft, G. (2015) Improving therapeutic relationships: Joint crisis planning for individuals with psychotic disorders. *Qualitative Health Research*, 25(12), 1637–1647.

Felton, A., Repper, J. and Avis, M. (2018) Therapeutic relationships, risk, and mental health practice. *International Journal of Mental Health Nursing*, 27(3), 1137–1148.

Flowers, M. and Hoult, J. (2008) Planning and implementing a local service. In S. Johnson, J. Needle, J. Bindman and G. Thornicroft (eds) *Crisis Resolution and Home Treatment in Mental Health*. Cambridge: Cambridge University Press, pp. 295–306.

Fook, J. (2004) Critical reflection and organisational learning and change: A case study. In N. Gould and M. Baldwin (eds) *Social Work, Critical Reflection and the Learning Organisation*. Aldershot: Ashgate Publishing, pp. 57–74.

Ford, R., Minghella, E., Chalmers, C., Hoult, J., Raftery, J. and Muijen, M. (2001) Cost consequences of home-based and in-patient-based acute psychiatric treatment: Results of an implementation study. *Journal of Mental Health*, 10(4), 467–476.

Gibson, S., Hamilton, S. and James, K. (2016) *Evaluation of the Crisis Care Concordat Implementation: Final Report*. Available at: https://www.crisiscareconcordat.org.uk/wp-content/uploads/2016/03/CCC-Evaluation_Report.pdf (accessed 1 June 2021).

Goh, C. and Agius, M. (2010) The stress-vulnerability model: How does stress impact on mental illness at the level of the brain and what are the consequences? *Psychiatria Danubina*, 22(2), 198–202.

Granello, D.H. (2010) A suicide crisis intervention model with 25 practical strategies for implementation. *Journal of Mental Health Counselling*, 32(3), 218–235.

Henwood, B.F., Derejko, K.S., Couture, J. and Padgett, D.K. (2015) Maslow and mental health recovery: A comparative study of homeless programs for adults with serious mental illness. *Administration and Policy in Mental Health*, 42(2), 220–228.

HM Government (2021) *Reforming the Mental Health Act*. Available at: https://www.gov.uk/government/consultations/reforming-the-mental-health-act/reforming-the-mental-health-act (accessed 1 April 2021).

HM Government and Mind (2014) Mental Health Crisis Care Concordat. Improving outcomes for people experiencing mental health crisis. Available at: https://assets.publishing.service.gov.uk/government/uploads/system/uploads/attachment_data/file/281242/36353_Mental_Health_Crisis_accessible.pdf (accessed 1 April 2021).

Hubbeling, D. and Bertram, R. (2012) Crisis resolution teams in the UK and elsewhere. *Journal of Mental Health*, 21(3), 285–295.

Hung, E.K., Binder, R.L., Fordwood, S.R., Hall, S.E., Cramer, R.J. and McNiel, D.E. (2012) A method for evaluating competency in assessment and management of suicide risk. *Academic Psychiatry: The Journal of the American Association of Directors of Psychiatric Residency Training and the Association for Academic Psychiatry*, 36(1), 23–28.

James, R.K. and Gilliland, B.E. (2016) *Crisis Intervention Strategies*, 8th edn. Boston, MA: Cengage Learning.

Johnson, S. (2013) Crisis resolution and home treatment teams: An evolving model. *Advances in Psychiatric Treatment*, 19(2), 115–123.

Johnson, S., Mason, O., Osborn, D., Milton, A., Henderson C., Marston, L., Ambler, G., Hunter, R., Pilning, S., ... and Lloyd-Evans, B. (2017) Randomised controlled trial of the clinical and cost-effectiveness of a peer-delivered self-management intervention to prevent relapse in crisis resolution team users: Study protocol. *British Medical Journal Open*, 7(10), 1–13.

Joiner, T.E. (2005) *Why People Die by Suicide*. Cambridge, MA: Harvard University Press.

Joiner, T.E., Ribeiro, J.D. and Silva, C. (2012) Nonsuicidal self-injury, suicidal behavior, and their co-occurrence as viewed through the lens of the interpersonal theory of suicide. *Current Directions in Psychological Science*, 21(5), 342–347.

Jones, M. (2020) Risk: A conversation worth having in mental health care? *Journal of Psychosocial Rehabilitation and Mental Health*, 7(1), 97–101.

Just, D., Palmier-Claus, J.E. and Tai, S. (2021) Positive risk management: Staff perspectives in acute mental health inpatient settings. *Journal of Advanced Nursing*, 77, 1899–1910.

Liu, J.J.W., Ein, N., Gervasio, J. and Vickers, K. (2019) The efficacy of stress reappraisal interventions on stress responsivity: A meta-analysis and systematic review of existing evidence. *PLoS One*, 14(2), 1–22.

Liu, Y., Pencheon, E., Hunter, R.M., Moncrieff, J. and Freemantle, N. (2018) Recruitment and retention strategies in mental health trials: A systematic review. *PloS One*, 13(8), 1–17.

Lloyd-Evans, B., Osborn, D., Marston, L., Lamb, D., Ambler, G., Hunter, R., Mason, O., Sullivan S., Henderson, C., … and Johnson, S. (2020) The CORE service improvement programme for mental health crisis resolution teams: Results from a cluster-randomised trial. *The British Journal of Psychiatry*, 216(6), 314–322.

Lloyd-Evans, B., Paterson, B., Onyett, S., Brown, E., Istead, H., Gray, R., Henderson, C. and Johnson, S. (2018) National implementation of a mental health service model: A survey of Crisis Resolution Teams in England. *International Journal of Mental Health Nursing*, 4(1), 214–226.

Lombardo, C., Santos, M., Van Bortel, T., Croos, R., Arensman, E. and Kar Ray, M. (2019) Decision-making in crisis resolution and home treatment teams: The AWARE framework. *BJPsych Bulletin*, 43(2), 61–66.

Ma, J., Batterham, P.J., Calear, A.L. and Han, J. (2016) A systematic review of the predictions of the Interpersonal-Psychological Theory of Suicidal Behavior. *Clinical Psychology Review*, 46, 34–45.

Mahomed, F. (2020) Addressing the problem of severe underinvestment in mental health and well-being from a human rights perspective. *Health and Human Rights*, 22(1), 35–49.

Maslow, A.H. (1954) *Motivation and Personality*. New York: Harper and Brothers.

McCrone, P., Johnson, S., Nolan, F., Pilling, S., Sandor, A., Hoult, J., McKenzie, N., Thompson, M. and Bebbington, P. (2009) Economic evaluation of a crisis resolution service: A randomised controlled trial. *Epidemiologia e Psichiatria Sociale*, 18(1), 54–58.

McKenna, B., Furness, T., Dhital, D., Ennis, G., Houghton, J., Lupson, C. and Toomey, N. (2014) Recovery-oriented care in acute inpatient mental health settings: An exploratory study. *Issues in Mental Health Nursing*, 35(7), 526–532.

Mental Health Act (1983) amended (2007). London: Department of Health. Available at: https://www.legislation.gov.uk/ukpga/2007/12/contents (accessed 20 April 2021).

Mental Health Foundation (2019) Crisis care. Available at: https://www.mentalhealth.org.uk/a-to-z/c/crisis-care#:~:text=A%20mental%20health%20crisis%20is,your%20physical%20or%20emotional%20wellbeing (accessed 3 May 2021).

Mental Health Foundation (2021) Stress. Available at: https://www.mentalhealth.org.uk/a-to-z/s/stress (accessed 3 May 2021).

Mind (2011) Listening to experience: An independent inquiry into acute and crisis mental healthcare. Available at: https://www.mind.org.uk/media-a/4377/listening_to_experience_web.pdf (accessed 4 April 2021).

Mind (2018) Crisis services and planning for a crisis: What are crisis teams? Available at: https://www.mind.org.uk/information-support/guides-to-support-and-services/crisis-services/crisis-teams-crhts/ (accessed 4 June 2021).

Morant, N., Lloyd-Evans, B., Lamb, D., Fullarton, K., Brown, E., Patterson, B., Istead, H., Kelly, K., Hindle, D., … and CORE Service User and Carer Working Groups (2017)

Crisis resolution and home treatment: Stakeholders' views on critical ingredients and implementation in England. *BMC Psychiatry*, 17(1), 1–13.

Morrissey, J., Doyle, L. and Higgins, A. (2018) Self-harm: From risk management to relational and recovery-oriented care. *The Journal of Mental Health Training, Education and Practice*, 13(1), 34–43.

Mulder, R., Newton-Howes, G. and Coid, J. (2016) The futility of risk prediction in psychiatry. *British Journal of Psychiatry*, 209(4), 271–272.

Murphy, S.M., Irving, C.B., Adams,C.E. and Waqar, M. (2015) Crisis intervention for people with severe mental illnesses. *Cochrane Database of Systematic Reviews*, 12, CD001087. Available at: https://doi.org/10.1002/14651858.CD001087.pub5

Newman-Taylor, K., Maguire, T. and Bowen, A. (2019) Why are we not measuring what matters in mental health in the UK? The case for routine use of recovery outcome measures. *Perspectives in Public Health*, 139(4), 181–183.

NHS (National Health Service) (2016) *The Five-Year Forward View for Mental Health*. Available at: https://www.england.nhs.uk/wp-content/uploads/2016/02/Mental-Health-Taskforce-FYFV-final.pdf (accessed 4 June 2021).

NHS (National Health Service) (2019a) *The NHS Long-Term Plan*. Available at: https://www.longtermplan.nhs.uk/wp-content/uploads/2019/08/nhs-long-term-plan-version-1.2.pdf (accessed 4 June 2021).

NHS (National Health Service) (2019b) *NHS Mental Health Implementation Plan 2019/20–2023/24*. Available at: https://www.longtermplan.nhs.uk/wp-content/uploads/2019/07/nhs-mental-health-implementation-plan-2019-20-2023-24.pdf (accessed 4 June 2021).

NHS (National Health Service) (2019c) Stress. Available at: https://www.nhs.uk/mental-health/feelings-symptoms-behaviours/feelings-and-symptoms/stress/ (accessed 4 June 2021).

NHS (National Health Service) (2020) Where to get urgent help for mental health. Available at: https://www.nhs.uk/mental-health/advice-for-life-situations-and-events/where-to-get-urgent-help-for-mental-health/ (accessed 4 June 2021).

NICE (National Institute for Clinical Excellence) (2011) *Service User Experience in Adult Mental Health: Improving the Experience of Care for People Using Adult NHS Mental Health Services*. NICE Clinical Guideline [CG136]. Available at: https://www.nice.org.uk/guidance/cg136/ifp/chapter/What-should-happen-in-a-crisis (accessed 4 June 2021).

NICE (National Institute for Clinical Excellence) (2017) *Managing Medicines for Adults Receiving Social Care in the Community*. NICE guideline [NG67]. Available at: https://www.nice.org.uk/guidance/ng67 (accessed 5 June 2021).

Nursing and Midwifery Council (2018) *The Code: Professional Standards of Practice and Behaviour for Nurses, Midwives and Nursing Associates*. Available at: http://www.nmc.org.uk/globalassets/sitedocuments/nmc-publications/revised-new-nmc-code.pdf (accessed 4 June 2021).

Oates, J., Drey, N. and Jones, J. (2017) 'Your experiences were your tools': How personal experience of mental health problems informs mental health nursing practice. *Journal of Psychiatric and Mental Health Nursing*, 24(7), 471–479.

Ogaku, P., McDonald A., Hakeem, S. and Sarfraz, A.M. (2018) Have crisis and home treatment teams become a second opinion or diagnostic service? *British Journal of Medical Practitioners*, 11(2), 1–4.

Olino, T.M., Mennies, R.J. and Wojcieszak, Z.K. (2020) Personality-stress vulnerability models. In E.P. Hayden and K.L. Harkness (eds) *The Oxford Handbook of Stress and Mental Health*. Oxford: Oxford University Press.

Onyett, S., Linde, K., Glover, G., Lloyd, S., Bradley, S. and Middleton, H. (2008) Implementation of crisis resolution/home treatment teams in England: National survey 2005–2006. *Psychiatric Bulletin*, 32, 374–377.

Paton, F., Wright, K., Ayre, N., Dare, C., Johnson, S., Lloyd-Evans, B., Simpson, A., Webber, M. and Meader, N. (2016) Improving outcomes for people in mental health crisis: A rapid synthesis of the evidence for available models of care. *Health Technology Assessment*, 20(3), 1–161.

Perkins, R. and Repper, J. (2016) Recovery versus risk? From managing risk to the co-production of safety and opportunity. *Mental Health and Social Inclusion*, 20(2), 101–109.

RCP (Royal College of Psychiatrists) (2016) Rethinking risk to others in mental health services (Council Report 201). Available at: https://www.rcpsych.ac.uk/docs/default-source/members/supporting-you/managing-and-assessing-risk/assessmentandman-agementrisktoothers.pdf?sfvrsn=a614e4f9_4 (accessed 11 May 2021).

RCP (Royal College of Psychiatrists) (2019) *Home Treatment Accreditation Scheme (HTAS) Standards for Home Treatment and Crisis Resolution Teams*, 4th edn. London: RCP. Available at: https://www.rcpsych.ac.uk/docs/default-source/improving-care/ccqi/quality-networks/htas/htas-standards-4th-edition.pdf?sfvrsn=a6908cbc_2 (accessed 11 May 2021).

RCP (Royal College of Psychiatrists) (2021) Country in the grip of a mental health crisis with children worst affected, new analysis finds. RCP Press Release. Available at: https://www.rcpsych.ac.uk/news-and-features/latest-news/detail/2021/04/08/country-in-the-grip-of-a-mental-health-crisis-with-children-worst-affected-new-analysis-finds (accessed 10 May 2021).

Recovery in the Bin (2019) Neorecovery: A survivor-led conceptualisation and critique. Available at: https://recoveryinthebin.org/2019/09/16/__trashed-2/ (accessed 13 April 2021).

Rethink (2020) Getting help in a crisis. Rethink Factsheet. Available at: https://www.rethink.org/advice-and-information/carers-hub/getting-help-in-a-crisis/ (accessed 13 April 2021).

Rethink (2021) Carer's hub. Available at: https://www.rethink.org/advice-and-information/carers-hub/ (accessed 11 May 2021).

Roberts, A.R. and Ottens, A.J. (2005) The seven-stage crisis intervention model: A road map to goal attainment, problem solving and crisis resolution. *Brief Treatment and Crisis Intervention*, 5, 329–339.

Royal College of General Practitioners (2017) 90 per cent of people with mental health problems cared for within primary care. Available at: https://www.rcgp.org.uk/clinical-and-research/about/clinical-news/2017/december/90-per-cent-of-people-with-mental-health-problems-cared-for-within-primary-care.aspx (accessed 11 May 2021).

Rudd, M.D., Joiner, T., Brown, G.K., Cukrowicz, K., Jobes, D.A., Silverman, M. and Cordero, L. (2009) Informed consent with suicidal patients: Rethinking risks in (and out of) treatment. *Psychotherapy: Theory, Research, Practice, Training*, 46(4), 459–468.

Sayer, A.M. (2017) Negotiating the interface between risk management and human rights-based care. In J. Warner, S. Stanford, E. Sharland and N.R. Heller (eds) *Beyond the Risk Paradigm in Mental Health Policy and Practice*. London: Palgrave.

Seery, M.D., Holman, E.A. and Silver, R.C. (2010) Whatever does not kill us: Cumulative lifetime adversity, vulnerability and resilience. *Journal of Personality and Social Psychology*, 99(6), 1025–1041.

Shaughnessy, L. (2015) Politics on the mind: Assessing the state of mental health after the election. *The Lancet: Psychiatry*, 2(4), 297–298.

Slade, M. (2009) *Personal Recovery and Mental Illness: A Guide for Mental Health Professionals (Values-Based Practice)*. Cambridge: Cambridge University Press.

Slade, M. and Longden, E. (2015) Empirical evidence about recovery and mental health. *BMC Psychiatry*, 15(285), 1–14.

Sreenath, S., Reddy, S., Tacchi, M. and Scott, J. (2010) Medication adherence in crisis. *Journal of Mental Health*, 19(5), 470–474.

Tees, Esk and Wear Valleys NHS Foundation Trust. (2021) Crisis resolution and intensive home treatment team (CRHT), urgent care services. Available at: https://www.tewv. nhs.uk/services/crisis-and-intensive-home-treatment-team/ (accessed 15 May 2021).

Tickle, A., Brown, D. and Hayward, M. (2014) Can we risk recovery? A grounded theory of clinical psychologists' perceptions of risk and recovery-oriented mental health services. *Psychology and Psychotherapy*, 87(1), 96–110.

University of Bristol (2020) *The Mental Wellbeing Toolbox: Handbook*. Available at: http://www.bris.ac.uk/vetscience/media/docs/mental_wellbeing.pdf (accessed 15 May 2021).

Van Heeringen, K. (2012) Stress-diathesis model of suicidal behavior. Available at: https://www.ncbi.nlm.nih.gov/books/NBK107203/ (accessed 15 May 2021).

Vos, J., Roberts, R. and Davies, J. (2019) *Mental Health in Crisis*. Los Angeles, CA: SAGE.

Vrshek-Schallhorn, S., Stroud, C.B., Mineka, S., Hammen, C., Zinbarg, R.E., Wolitzky-Taylor, K. and Craske, M.G. (2015) Chronic and episodic interpersonal stress as statistically unique predictors of depression in two samples of emerging adults. *Journal of Abnormal Psychology*, 124(4), 918–932.

Walsh, F. (2007) Traumatic loss and major disasters: Strengthening family and community resilience. *Family Process*, 46, 207–227.

Werbeloff, N., Chang, C.K., Broadbent, M., Hayes, J.F., Stewart, R. and Osborn, D.P.J. (2017) Admission to acute mental health services after contact with crisis resolution and home treatment teams: An investigation in two large mental health-care providers. *The Lancet Psychiatry*, 4(1), 49–56.

WHO (World Health Organisation) (2019) Mental health in emergencies: Factsheet. Available at: https://www.who.int/news-room/fact-sheets/detail/mental-health-in-emergencies (accessed 15 May 2021).

Zubin, J. and Spring, B. (1977) Vulnerability: A new view of schizophrenia. *Journal of Abnormal Psychology*, 86, 103–126.

4 Policing the mental health crisis

Anne Eason, Rob Starr and Matt Gaunt

The chapter considers the role of the police in supporting a person experiencing a mental health crisis. Like paramedics, the police are commonly the frontline helping professionals involved in crisis scenarios. Situations involve assisting an individual at immediate risk of ending their life, who may be a risk to others, or appears to be experiencing a mental disorder requiring a mental health assessment. Despite the police force striving, when possible, to have therapeutic encounters with a person in need, problems exist with understanding mental distress, alongside concerns that police involvement may lead to criminalising the individual. This chapter aims to contribute to the ongoing debate about the role of the police on these occasions. Rather than providers of a 'sticking plaster' strategy that neither benefits the individual nor the community, it will be suggested the police have a role with wider collaborative strategies, working closely with service partners who have the skills and knowledge to instigate cohesive and effective crisis care.

Introduction

There has long been a synergy between those suffering with mental health issues and their interactions with police and the wider criminal justice sector. According to Mental Health First Aid (MHFA) England (2020), more than 30 per cent of the public believe that those with a mental health diagnosis commit violent offences in the community, yet statistics show they are more likely to be a victim of crime than a perpetrator. MHFA (2020) state that 80–90 per cent of those who attempt or complete suicide, have a mental health issue, sometimes undiagnosed. In some constabularies such as Avon and Somerset, a south-western region of the UK, specific measures have been taken by the police in conjunction with the Fire Service, the Ambulance Service, the County Council and other allied sector agencies, to reduce accessibility to popular suicide locations such as the Bristol Avon Gorge (Pitts, 2018). Most detentions actioned by police in England and Wales are for the prevention of suicide, and the lack of mental health support services has resulted in front-line officers often bearing the brunt of intervening at such times of crisis (Warrington, 2019).

The criminal justice sector is overwhelmed with an offending community that have or are experiencing mental health problems. Together for Mental Wellbeing (2020) reports that over 70 per cent of the prison population have some form of mental health issue. Moreover, the Prison Reform Trust (2020) suggests that most of those who have fatally self-harmed in prison were known to have some type of mental health problem. In a recent HMIP (Her Majesty's Inspectorate Probation) inspection report of the Probation Service (Sirdifield and Brooker, 2020), only speculative figures have been proposed in regard to how many of those offenders under community supervision have some form of mental health problem, suggesting many suffer co-morbidity and a high number of dual-diagnoses often triggered by substance misuse. Several studies also concluded that personality disorders were the highest among those supervised by probation, including Knauer, Walker and Roberts (2017), and a further study undertaken by Phillips, Padfield and Gelsthorpe (2018) suggests the suicide rate for this group of offenders is 'nine times higher than in the general population' (Sirdifield and Brooker, 2020, p. 4). With such high numbers, criminal justice agencies, including the public, private and third sector, have had to diversify their practice to give a pragmatic response to support these offenders, particularly with the Covid-19 pandemic creating a vacuum for intensifying mental health problems and significantly impacting on the way in which services operate.

While police officers have contact with people experiencing mental health crisis in a variety of contexts, the primary legislation to care for those believed to require treatment comes from Section 136 of the Mental Health Act (MHA, 1983). Broadly, this gives police officers the power to remove a person to a place of safety if it appears that they are suffering from a mental disorder, and are in need of immediate care and control (MHA 1983, s. 136). This gives the police significant power to deprive a person of their liberty to seek further assessment by mental health professionals, though not the power to 'section'; the role of the police is to facilitate assessment. Another gateway for accessing mental health services may be an arrest for a criminal offence, with The Police and Criminal Evidence Act (PACE, 1984) placing a duty on the custody officer to ensure that a person receives clinical attention if they appear to be suffering from a mental disorder (PACE Act 1984, Code C, 9.5). 'Detention' under the Act is not defined, but this could lead to the person being deemed unfit to be detained in police custody, and instead detained by an approved mental health professional under section and transferred to hospital.

Thus, in this ongoing struggle to find more effective and empathic ways of managing those with mental health issues (especially coping with the recent Covid-19 restrictions and the increasing numbers of those affected by it), there has been a concerted drive to take a more joined-up approach to crisis management in the community (Kirubarajan *et al.*, 2018; Rodgers *et al.*, 2019). Responding to austerity measures that have depleted the emergency services and their agency partners, innovative models of working have been designed and deployed to avert the tragedy of suicide and divert those with mental health needs away from criminality and their vulnerability to criminal victimhood.

This chapter explores the role of the police in their interactions with these members of the public, as a single agency and as part of a multi-agency model, that explores the effectiveness of current legislative interventions.

The current landscape

Interprofessional working is central to the public protection agenda and the role of the criminal justice sector, including the police (Fox, 2019; Nash, 2010). Policing involves what Jones, Newburn and Reiner (2017) describe as 'a miscellany of tasks', an instantaneous response to stakeholder demand, whether public or state, to keep the peace and protect those who are vulnerable from the risk of serious harm and/or social conflict. Formalised through the Criminal Justice and Court Services Act 2000 S. 67 and 68, the police are actively engaged in multi-agency working, including information sharing through various forums such as MAPPA (Multi-Agency Public Protection Arrangements) and MARAC (Multi-Agency Risk Assessment Conferences), discussed further in Chapter 6 (College of Policing, 2018; Loveday and Roberts, 2019; Nash, 2010). The College of Policing (2018) promotes the idea of police being proactive in the joined-up approach to managing high risk of harm offenders and coordinated assessment as an effective method in the management thus and reduction of risk. However, it is not just offenders with whom the police have contact when there is a mental health emergency, in terms of response (outlined in Chapter 3).

As first responders, the police are often confronted with individuals who are in crisis but have no forensic history and are not perhaps known to any mental health agency. Those individuals often fall into the high risk of harm category outlined in multi-agency guidance (Gough, 2019) and warrant the joined-up working of multi-disciplinary teams in a holistic approach to their assessment and management (Winstone, 2019). Winstone suggests that while the multi-disciplinary approach is likely the most successful for reducing the incidence of harm to self and/or others by those in crisis, this can only be achieved through a strategy that is flexible and collaborative, pointing out 'there is not a one-stop-shop for solutions' (2019, p. 245) that will fit all scenarios. The police need support from those who are trained in assessing and engaging individuals in crisis, whether offenders or not, to understand and assist in de-escalating very complex needs.

The College of Policing and Association of Chief Police Officers, along with other public sector national organisations, signed the Mental Health Crisis Care Concordat in 2014 to assist in the improvement of responses to those with mental ill-health and as part of this multi-disciplinary approach that can support harm reduction (HM Government and Mind, 2014). The government guidance recognised the inappropriate use of police cells to detain those in crisis due to the lack of specialist services and that the police were neither skilled, nor should they be, to provide the type of professional support that is required. In a similar vein to how multi-agency forums such as MAPPA or MARAC operate in the management of high risk of harm offenders or protecting high risk victims, the Concordat offers a strategy of multi-disciplinary cooperation to provide a coordinated approach to supporting those with mental health issues. The role of the police within this forum is not, however, clear-cut.

Unlike the public protection arrangements via MAPPA and other stated multi-agency forums that are an accepted part of everyday policing practice, the location of the police within the Mental Health Crisis Care Concordat (HM Government and Mind, 2014) is somewhat less concrete. As discussed by our paramedic cousins in Chapter 5, the police are often part of a firefighting duo that merely provide a sticking plaster for an austerity-ridden mental health service that is unable to respond in a timely manner to those in crisis, and of which there have been increasing numbers in recent years (Wondemaghen, 2021).

The use of police cells as alternatives to places that can provide the health-based care necessary to de-escalate the risk of harm has resulted in the police function of the Concordat as that of a 'stop-gap' for not only detention but of fielding other behavioural issues, such as nuisance calls. The White Paper, 'Reforming the Mental Health Act' (UK Government, 2021, p. 11) states that the NHS (National Health Service) Long-Term Plan seeks to make redundant the use of police cells through the enhancement of crisis intervention services and, during the period 2018/19, the majority of those detained under Section 136 were indeed placed in health-based places as opposed to police custody.

Nevertheless, for those who do not reach health-based places, the custody officer is expected, as shown in case study 4.1, to be able to conduct continuous and accurate risk assessments to prevent harm and often without any background information (Leese and Russell, 2017). Leese and Russell's study of vulnerability and risk in police custody reported officer concerns around their responsibility: 'it's a massive challenge for the police ... because we are seen as a jack of all trades' (2017, p. 277). However, little training exists to prepare police officers for the significant numbers of mentally unwell detainees and the associated complexities of illness and criminality.

Case study 4.1   Abdul

Abdul is a 19-year-old man who lives with his mother. Two months ago, Abdul was removed from university because of his aggressive behaviour, which resulted in a criminal conviction for assaults, a public order offence and drugs. Since returning home Abdul has been verbally aggressive and abusive to his mother, which has been escalating quickly. He has told his mother many times that he wishes she was dead, and has sent her a letter, telling her that he was going to kill her the next day. Abdul has refused to see his GP and has never been treated for mental health conditions.

Abdul's mother is so concerned that she calls the police. The police find a note in his bedroom detailing how he will tie her up and kill her in the garage, and in the garage is a chair with rope and knives. When booked into custody,

Abdul is seen by a nurse, who assesses, although distressed, he is fit to be detained and interviewed. Officers attempt to build a rapport and ask about the letter sent to his mother. The officers recognise the need for a gentle discussion, which achieves the goal of gathering information but does not distress Abdul further. The outcome was a charge with Abdul threatening to kill his mother, and during the court process mental health assessments are conducted. Abdul pleads guilty and receives a hospital order.

Questions continue to be raised about the role of the police within this facet of the multi-agency landscape. When releasing their Authorised Professional Practice (APP), the College of Policing Lead for Mental Health stated:

Police are not mental health professionals and our aim is to deal with any offences committed and protect the public from harm. It will continue to be the responsibility of health and welfare agencies to assist those in mental health crisis.

(College of Policing, 2016)

The 2018 report, 'Policing and Mental Health: Picking up the Pieces', by Her Majesty's Inspectorate of Constabulary and Fire and Rescue Services (HMIC-FRS) goes further still, stating 'we have grave concerns about whether the police should be involved in responding to mental health problems to the degree they are' (HMICFRS, 2018a, p. 3). HMICFRS describe the mental health system as broken, and that other agencies should stop relying as heavily on the police. This damning assessment from a regulatory body independent of the police themselves calls into question the structure of current multi-agency practices; while the premise of working together is admirable, without resourcing a nationally agreed structure to support this approach, police will continue to be used inappropriately as a lead agency in circumstances outside of their primary role and knowledge spectrum.

Mental health training

Current training for police in mental health is limited. The mental health APP as set out by the College of Policing (2016) is provided via the NCALT (National Centre for Applied Learning Technologies) learning environment. Set up specifically to support the police forces of England and Wales in the delivery of e-learning courses, the NCALT forum houses the mental health APP which focuses on how police should respond to effectively interact with those suffering with mental health issues and other developmental conditions. Set within the parameters of the legislative and policy framework comprising the Policing and Crime Act 2017 and the Mental Health Act 1983, the guidance includes advice on how to detect, detain and assess those individuals and protect them and the public from any risk of harm. However, this training relies upon the police officer not only to undertake it when directed, but to also meaningfully engage with the material.

The point raised about engagement is significant. A study by Honess (2020) exploring police officer attitudes towards mandatory e-learning training, particularly via NCALT, found that the majority of officers were neither motivated to complete it nor was it an effective method of learning. This suggests that the little input police officers do receive about mental health is neither reliable in terms of comprehension or, indeed, that it has been anything more than just a tick box exercise to satisfy targeted performance indicators rather than being usefully understood and applied to everyday dealings with mental health incidents. Most participants in the research preferred a more blended approach that opened up opportunities to discuss, debate and clarify meanings, of behaviours and understandings of very complex situations. In addition, there is no formal requirement for serving officers to undertake any continuous professional development in relation to mental health over and above College of Policing-dictated e-learning packages. For some individual officers, their knowledge may have been gained long before current guidance and case law came into effect. In the case of the APP, it is possible that many officers will not have read it or kept themselves up-to-date with amendments.

With the latest professionalisation routes to training new recruits, including the PCDA (Police Constable Degree Apprenticeship), there is much more opportunity for interactive learning about the complexities of mental health and the legislative framework within which police officers have to operate. Although the curriculum is still governed by the College of Policing (2021) in the PEQF (Policing Education Qualifications Framework), collaborative delivery of training with higher education institutes means that at least some of the learning will take a more blended approach (Honess, 2020). This may satisfy some of the concerns raised about pure e-learning packages and also offer opportunities for specialist input and conversational learning.

Nevertheless, the curriculum is condensed, time-limited and although pedagogically designed, is still arguably constrained and does not form part of any CPD (continuous professional development) package. Some forces have developed additional handbooks, digital apps and checklists for officers to refer to when they encounter an individual with mental health needs (HMICFRS, 2018b), often with multi-agency links for support, particularly with those with multiple diagnoses. But with a limited legislative and policy framework through which the police are able to manage incidents of crisis, the need for urgent revision of powers and indeed roles and resources in the reform of the Mental Health Act (UK Government, 2021), we would argue, is a necessity. The inevitable consequences of a care system stripped back to the minimum is bound to result in a piecemeal system where some great work is being undertaken but much more is left to services with little specialist training, such as the police, in the challenges presented by those living with psychological and psychiatric difficulties.

Implementing Section 136

The role of the police in England and Wales, indeed in many areas of the world, is to keep the peace. In England and Wales, those who hold 'the office of Constable' take an oath in the presence of a Magistrate in which they swear to: 'cause the [Queen's] peace to be kept and preserved and [to] prevent all offences against people and property' (Police Federation, 2018). The word 'peace', in a policing context, is a nebulous one replete with many nuanced meanings. It can require a myriad of responses and interactions, from talking to young people about the dangers of illicit drugs, to the donning of public order equipment in order to face a rioting crowd, who most certainly are not being peaceful. A violent offender committing an offence towards a person such as an assault or criminal damage to property will, it is suggested, be breaking the Queen's peace. Section 24 of The Police and Criminal Evidence Act 1984 (PACE) provides a constable with the power to arrest without warrant anyone whom they have 'reasonable grounds to suspect of being guilty of [committing] it' (Home Office, 2019). The *Oxford English Dictionary* provides a definition of the word arrest, the sentiment of which still holds legally true despite the outdated language: 'to restrain a man of his liberty, obliging him to be obedient to the law'. To note, for a person suspected of breaching the Queen's law, legal 'restraint' is the consequence: a person's liberty is taken from them upon being detained by a police officer.

In England and Wales, even those not suspected of committing an offence can also be legally detained by a police officer. This scenario could very easily be the position in which a person suffering from a mental disorder could find themselves. A person who is ill can have their liberty taken from them simply because they appear, to a constable, to be mentally unwell and there is a concern for safety. As outlined in Chapters 3 and 6, Section 136 of the Mental Health Act 1983 (MHA) states:

> If a person appears to a constable to be suffering from mental disorder and to be in an immediate need of care and control, the constable may, if he thinks it necessary to do so in the interests of that person or for the protection of other persons –
>
> (a) remove that person to a place of safety within the meaning of Section 135 or
>
> (b) if the person is already at a place of safety within the meaning of that section, keep the person at that place or remove the person to another place of safety.

The above legislation permits a person to be detained for a period of 24 hours. This begins when the person has been removed to a place of safety, with the time commencing when they arrive at that place. It is important to note that in such cases, the person detained under the Mental Health Act has not committed a criminal offence. Their detention is purely based upon the assessment of a police officer that they appear to be ill: 'suffering from mental disorder' and they pose a risk of harm.

There is the potential for significant impact on a member of the public who is detained under s. 136 and this is heightened when the individual must be physically transferred to a secure location, referred to in the legislation as a 'place of safety' and which for some, will be police cells until the appropriate specialist is available to assess them. To a person without forensic history, one who has not committed an offence, such an environment may appear to be anything but safe. Legislatively, then, what is deemed 'a place of safety'? It is defined in Section 135 of the Mental Health Act 1983 as being: 'a residential accommodation provided by a local social services authority ... a hospital as defined by this Act, a police station, an independent hospital or care home for mentally disordered persons or any other suitable place'.

No part of a police station can be viewed as a place of safety for children and for adults only in extreme circumstances, such as if a person poses an imminent risk of harm or death to themselves or another (Angiolini, 2017). It is not for the officer on the street to decide what constitutes a 'place of safety' as this is a matter for agencies such as health and social care, but the officer does have a lot of other decisions to make: Does the person *appear* to be suffering from a *mental disorder* and to be in *immediate* need of care and control? Are they a danger to themselves or anyone else either by the person's actions or the environment? If they are, then immediate action must be taken and using police cells may be the only available option.

If we consider the power of arrest provided by Section 24 PACE, as detailed above, when attending an incident, an officer must assess the situation in order to arrive at an objective legal threshold that allows them to formulate suspicion before detaining an individual. While each situation is different, and therefore suspicion is always, to a degree, a subjective position to be arrived at by the officer, student constables do receive extensive procedural and legal training upon which they can draw in order to reach a decision to arrest. In relation to Section 136 MHA (1983), the parameters set within the legislation are not so legally rigorous. If we look at the wording of s. 136, then legally a person can be detained solely upon how their actions 'appear', a word that does not feature in legal guidance or is quantified in officer training. In the case of mental health legislation, therefore, subjectivity is predicated upon how a person's actions 'appear' to an officer.

The contexts in which non-mental health-trained officers must assess an individual to determine the appropriateness of s. 136 are specific. The Mental Health Act states that Section 136 cannot be used if the location of an incident is within 'any house, flat or room where that person, or any other person is living', including certain outside spaces connected with that dwelling, for example, 'any yard, garden, garage, or outhouse that is connected with the house, flat, or room'. So, while seemingly giving power to officers to intervene at times of crisis, s. 136 specifically prevents officers acting inside a dwelling. This is clearly problematic as officers frequently attend incidents, as in case study 4.2, in which individuals in crisis are inside their own homes, although this can, in part, be mitigated by Section 135 of the Mental Health Act. Provision is made for an Approved Mental Health Professional (AMHP, see Chapter 6) to apply to a Justice of the Peace for a warrant allowing an officer, accompanied by an AMHP and registered medical practitioner, to gain entry and transport the person to a place of safety for a Mental Health Act assessment (Mental Health Act 1983, s. 135 (1)).

Case study 4.2   John

John is a 46-year-old man, who lives alone. Police have been called by John at 3 a.m. to his home address, telling the control room staff that he had a knife and wanted to end his own life. John has called the police 14 times before to similar incidents. John has previously had a stroke and has mobility problems.

The attending officers can see that John has no injuries. John is in the sitting room watching home videos, which he says are of his wife and children before they left him. He appears distressed. John asks for help because he wants to write a suicide note to his family and due to the stroke is no longer able to do so. John is adamant that he will kill himself that night.

Officers contact the out-of-hours crisis team who cannot attend, telling officers that John has made similar claims previously, but it has been found he is not at high risk of suicide. The officers present are concerned about John but have no legal power to intervene in this situation and feel ill-prepared to determine his risk.

While Section 135 appears to bridge the gap with s. 136, practical challenges may impact on using the legislation, in what are often volatile and dynamic situations. For example, police may be called at night to a person harming themselves with a knife. The mention of a knife would see police as the primary responders, presented with a situation in which they have no legal power to intervene, resulting in a dilemma when the officer must balance their duty to preserve life with their inability to lawfully act. Furthermore, the s. 135 warrant, which provides the potential solution, may not guarantee the emergency support needed, especially 'out of hours'. It is these situations which have caused such difficulties for the police, unable to appropriately judge risk due to a lack of expertise in mental health, but also unable to simply leave the situation to those professionals who can. In these circumstances, the event would likely unfold very publicly, potentially heightening the risk factors both for the individual requiring assistance and the officers who are attempting to assist them (Edwards and Kotera, 2020).

Police officers have often used other legislation in lieu of the Mental Health Act, in particular, the Common Law power to prevent a Breach of the Peace and Section 5 of the Mental Capacity Act 2005. The Mental Capacity Act 2005 (MCA) provides a statutory framework for individuals (aged 16 or older) who lack capacity to make specific decisions for themselves, or who have capacity but want to make preparations for a time in the future when they may lack the ability to make such decisions. The MCA does not apply to any one specific agency or individual but Chapter 6 of the Code of Practice (MCA Codes of Practice, 2007), issued in relation to this legislation, outlines when the police, and other agencies, can detain, restrain and take a person to hospital. Significantly, the MCA does apply, unlike s. 136 MHA, to private premises.

The MCA is most likely to be used by police officers in an emergency situation when a person, who is lacking mental capacity, is at risk or may suffer harm if action is not taken, for example, a person attempting or threatening suicide, victims of serious assaults or casualties of major incidents. As the MCA Code of Practice 2007, para. 6.35 states: 'In emergencies, it will almost always be in the person's best interests to give urgent treatment without delay.' The use of the word 'almost' provides a degree of discretion for any agencies involved in the potential use of the MCA because at all times a person is deemed to have capacity to make decisions unless a lack of capacity is established. The MCA provides for officers to take immediate decisions that 'relate to containing, controlling and potentially restraining an individual who lacks the capacity to make the decision in question for themselves, while awaiting further input or direction from a health or social care professional' (College of Policing, 2016). In such a situation, officers can use reasonable force to protect and control a person who does not have the mental capacity to protect themselves. However, while the police are empowered to act under this legislation, case law has shown that using this instead of powers conferred by the Mental Health Act is unlawful.

In the case of *Sessay vs South London and Maudsley NHS Trust (R (Sessay) v South London and Maudsley NHS Foundation Trust* [2011] EWHC 2617), police officers entered Sessay's residence and detained her, believing she was mentally disordered. Officers then took her to a mental health hospital ward known as the '136 Suite', justifying their actions by stating that they were acting under Section 5 of the Mental Capacity Act. The courts held that the actions taken were unlawful, and that the Mental Capacity Act could not be used by officers to remove a person suffering from a mental disorder to a place of safety. Importantly, the judgment found that any gap in the Mental Health Act 1983 was for Parliament to fill rather than for officers to circumvent.

The complexities of the discussed legislation, the Mental Health Act and the Mental Capacity Act, and lack of mental health support, place officers in volatile situations when trying to keep an individual and community safe from harm. Officer training has already been covered in the chapter but a phrase that resonates with its limitations is that of Teplin and Pruett (1992), whose article title describes American police officers as being 'street-corner psychiatrist(s)'. Required to work in public places, a 'streetcorner', as well as in private spaces, and make decisions without the assistance of those with specialist knowledge, i.e. the 'psychiatrist[s]', the hint of irony conveyed by the term highlights the lack of training British officers receive in identifying mental health disorders.

Good practice with mental health crisis

Michael Lipsky claims that public sector workers, such as police officers, are often required to exercise their professional discretion in the wide range of incidents they attend, making high-level decisions 'on the spot and totally focused upon the individual' (1980, p. 8) with often little information, time, or specialist resources to hand (1980, p. xi). Officers are often required to make decisions in the moment, based not upon an objective set of circumstances, those from which criminal suspicion could be derived, but rather upon psychological and/or physical symptoms a person 'appears' to be exhibiting to a non-medically trained police constable, in a dynamic and potentially dangerous environment. In this respect, Teplin and Pruett's (1992) description of police officers as 'streetcorner psychiatrists' is particularly insightful as it captures that sense of immediacy, stress and potential danger for all parties; factors often present when called to an incident.

The above does not suggest police officers are without resources to call upon when faced with an emergency involving a person experiencing a mental health crisis. It is recognised there are medical professionals who work with police officers in triage teams but they are not on duty in all force areas every moment of each day. Also, as to be expected, they are a limited resource and so officers cannot always rely on them to attend an incident even when on duty, due to the demand put upon their skills. According to the Office for National Statistics (2019), in 2019, there were 5,316 suicides in England and Wales – that is more than 15 a day – with many attempts also made. London's Metropolitan Police Service, the largest force in Britain, receives a call related to mental health every four minutes (HMICFRS, 2018) while Andy Marsh, Avon and Somerset Constabulary's Chief Constable, has stated that his force receives 100 calls a day related to mental health incidents, 16 per cent of their daily total (Postans, 2019). In respect of the national perspective, we can see a year-on-year increase in s. 136 detentions, where in the year ending March 2020, there were 31,825; a 2 per cent increase on the same period from 2019 (Home Office, 2020).

With such high rates of mental health-related reports, in October 2019, Avon and Somerset Constabulary (ASC) introduced a process whereby police officers, Police Community Support Officers (PCSOs) and police staff, in addition to their day-to-day role, also undertake the task of mental health tactical advisors (MHTAs). These individuals are available to officers either through their force radio network or on the telephone and are there to provide support in mental health incidents. The MHTAs have an in-depth understanding of mental health law, together with the relevant codes of practice, and as such can offer advice to officers who are at an incident and assisting a member of the public who could be in crisis. They are not, however, clinicians or indeed in place to act as a pseudo-clinician, but they are able to review the history of any contact the person may have had with ASC and to gain information from other agencies, for example, the NHS or Social Services, and if appropriate in the context of the incident, a member of the person's family. The availability of the MHTA resource is not a 24/7 facility, however. Furthermore, not all staff in ASC's control rooms are trained MHTAs and due to workload, among other reasons, may not be available when officers need support. Nevertheless, availability of such staff aside, the presence and use of MHTAs within a police control room are both a source of support for officers and by extension also for members of the public who may be experiencing a mental health crisis.

While initiatives such as the MHTA instituted by ASC are available remotely to officers, in 2013, a geographically wider initiative, and one more closely connected to patrol officers, was put in place in England by the Department of Health. The street triage scheme involves dedicated mental health professionals working collaboratively with the police, attending scenes and offering appropriate interventions tailored to the needs of the person in crisis. In doing so, the problems of inappropriate 'places of safety' and delays in medical treatment can be averted and the police officers can go about their crime-fighting duties.

While the triage scheme is potentially useful to those in crisis, and to the officer who will be guided and assisted by a healthcare professional, it is not without its problems. Mental health practitioners must adhere to ethical considerations, one of which is consent. Having previously discussed s. 136, we know that legislation allows officers to detain a person where there is a risk of significant harm and commission a professional to assess/treat them. But in most circumstances, individuals have the right to choose if they wish to interact with mental health services. A concern raised by Fiona Sweeney is 'that service users may feel somewhat obliged or forced to speak to professionals in fear or doubt around what may result if they refuse' (Sweeney, 2015, p. 677). Sweeney believes there are ethical considerations around officers attending such incidents as their presence may provoke unwarranted legal consequences should the individual not wish to engage. This is an area, Sweeney suggests, that needs attention, just as are the broader issues about training, or the lack thereof, highlighted earlier.

Sweeney's (2015) identification of the ethical considerations of consent is but one potentially problematic issue around street triage. A second is availability. Due to limited resources, not every police officer will have access to street triage services. A national survey of mental health trusts sought to gather information detailing street triage services, including determining officers' experiences and views of the service within a specific force area Thames Valley Police (TVP). Some 98 per cent of TVP officers who responded to the survey stated the 'service was highly beneficial' and that officers were 'overwhelmingly supportive of street triage' (Kirubarajan *et al.*, 2018, p. 256). This survey found the service was only available in 70 per cent of England with variations throughout as to the availability of services: '[h]ours of operation vary, although usually with an emphasis on evenings, night-times and weekends with little or no cover during the daytime' (p. 256). This lack of service availability was the one area of street triage provision that was criticised by officers, the majority of whom would like to see it 'available 24/7' (p. 257).

As statistics discussed earlier illustrate, mental health incidents form a large part of the police's work. It is often the police who 'fulfil the role of gatekeeper' (Kane *et al.*, 2017, p. 2) when it comes to deciding if a person with a mental health disorder should enter the mental health or criminal justice system. Two methods by which such individuals are provided with appropriate help have been discussed, MHTAs and street triage, with both receiving overwhelming support from officers. Two other interventions are also available to some police areas: Liaison and Diversion (L and D) together with Crisis Intervention Teams (CITs). L and D seeks to divert individuals at the earliest point they enter the criminal justice system (CJS). Mental health-trained staff are embedded in police custody suites or in courts in order to assess and refer individuals for whom mental health services outside of the CJS may be appropriate. Of course, this process is post-arrest and so will not assist officers at incidents but crucially it is a means by which a person experiencing mental health problems can access medical help rather than be placed into the justice system.

Kane *et al.* (2017, p. 3) mention CITs as a fourth intervention, one developed in 1988 following the fatal shooting of a man suffering from a history of drug abuse and mental illness by a Memphis police officer. This intervention is carried out by specially trained officers who work alone, or with healthcare professionals, in instances where individuals with mental health problems require help. The aim of the programme is to increase safety for all parties and to divert a person from the justice system towards the mental health system. A study in the United States by Taheri (2016) found CITs to have no impact on the arrests of individuals with mental illness or on officer safety, however:

> the null effects of CITs on arrest and use of force outcomes may or may not be explained by the types of evaluations currently available, and should be examined further when more research is available. However, they do suggest that these programs are promising in some studies and on average do not do any harm to the populations they set out to serve.
>
> (Taheri, 2016, p. 92)

Further research is clearly needed to examine the efficacy of CITs generally, and specifically within the United Kingdom, but in 2020 the College of Policing reviewed Taheri's article, agreeing with the author's findings. The fact that in CITs an officer is encouraged to collaborate with other agencies to arrive at the best outcome for the individual, one predicated as much upon care as incarceration, is an aim the College of Policing, not just the organisation but those for whom this term is a professional abbreviation, must strive to achieve.

With limited powers and mental health knowledge, the question of why the police are called upon to engage with people in crisis is worth exploring. As with all public sector agencies, a review takes place when a death or serious injury occurs which leads to public and media scrutiny of police performance. While this is not exclusive to those suffering with mental health issues, there are damning reports of police heavy-handedness, particularly when using physical restraint in their effort to gain control of an individual whom they assess as a threat, whether to self or others, as seen in the case of Leon Briggs who died in police custody (Angiolini, 2017).

In Angiolini's report on deaths and serious incidents in police custody, the author sets out the problems encountered by police officers as the first point of contact for concerned members of the public, when faced with an individual in crisis. Police forces in England and Wales are subject to scrutiny from a variety of sources. In addition to the courts (criminal, civil and coroner), individual incidents may be subject to investigation by the Independent Office for Police Complaints (IOPC), or Safeguarding Adults Reviews as defined by the Care Act 2014. These reviews all play a part in understanding how failings may have occurred, and instilling a culture of learning for the future. Independent inspection of police practices is completed by HMICFRS, who review the effectiveness and efficiency of forces, with their principal role being 'to promote improvements in policing and fire and rescue services to make everyone safer' (HMICFRS, 2018b). In their most recent report examining policing and mental health in 2018, HMICFRS found the police response to be 'generally supportive, considerate and compassionate' (HMICFRS, 2018a, p. 3). The report describes the police as generally having strong leadership and governance, with individual officers able to identify those who need support. Despite this, problems persist with inconsistent training, a lack of understanding of the demand placed upon forces, and most forces do not seek the views of people who have mental health problems (HMICFRS, 2018a).

Research by Pettitt *et al.* (2013) addressed the lack of a voice for those experiencing mental health problems within the criminal justice system, examining perceptions of the police and wider criminal justice agencies. The research focused on victimisation and engagement with the criminal justice system, rather than in relation to the use of s. 136 powers, but highlighted some key issues in the way these people had been treated by the police. Experiences were mixed, with participants in the study frequently reporting both good and bad experiences. There was a perception from some that experiencing mental health problems might be used as a reason for the police to disbelieve them, along with a fear of being 'sectioned' for reporting crimes. Some respondents felt there was discrimination in their treatment within the criminal justice system, with a decline in their mental health following interactions with police, suggesting empathy and understanding were seen as essential qualities for officers. This research highlights the impact that individual officers can have, with good and bad experiences proving to have an influence; the success of policing those experiencing mental ill-health is, at least in part, in the hands of the police themselves.

Conclusion

Policing in the twenty-first century is significantly more complex than in previous decades with increasingly higher numbers of the community, including the offending community, suffering a mental health crisis. Suicides, self-harm and psychotic episodes now account for a significant proportion of incidents attended by police (Home Office, 2020) and with Phillips, Padfield and Gelsthorpe (2018) reporting that suicide rates in those being supervised by probation services are nine times higher than those of the general population, it is not surprising that incidents involving this cohort are increasing. But what is police responsibility in terms of managing these situations? The primary role of police officers is to detect and deter crime and criminality, protect the public and work with others in the prevention and reduction of crime-harm (Gough, 2019). This of course will involve those in mental health crisis, however, the limitation of powers often renders their efforts to enact their role unachievable and, where their efforts fail, open to governmental, public and media scrutiny.

Given the frequency of police attendance of incidents where mental health is a contributory factor, one question particularly comes to the fore: why is training for police officers so limited? Despite their repeated interactions with members of the public who are suffering a mental health episode, that many police officers still feel they lack the training to adequately deal with such incidents (HMICFRS, 2018a) is of grave concern. As we have highlighted above, student police officers are currently trained within a classroom environment, following the PEQF curriculum designed by the College of Policing (2021). This includes what legislation is applicable to detain a person suffering from a mental health problem, the powers they can use and/or what constitutes a 'place of safety', but they do not undertake detailed training in how to assess a person's mental state prior to using their lawful powers, arguably putting both the officer and individual at risk.

Operational policing frequently relies upon professional discretion and the officers' overall understanding of the situation features significantly in the decision-making process. In situations when mental health is part of the incident dynamic, limited knowledge or understanding of mental health diagnoses and the most effective techniques in which to interact with those in crisis creates understandable tensions, poorly thought-out strategies and the potential for criminalisation of an individual who just needs treatment (Leese and Russell, 2017; Teplin and Pruett, 1992). The officers' assessment of the behaviour they are faced with and the need for responses such as restraint or detention, is thus born out of their interpretation of the restrictive legislative framework in that unique situation; a street-level implementation (Lipsky, 1980) that may or may not result in the best outcome.

The current criminal justice landscape supports the holistic approach of interprofessional working to manage those considered most dangerous and those at highest risk of harm. The triage scheme uses this joined-up methodology bringing specialists to the incident rather than removing the individual to what often constitutes an environment not conducive to their needs. Indeed, often an environment, such as police cells, is where their condition may worsen. This practice was reportedly well received by officers (Kirubarajan *et al.*, 2018) and seemingly effective for mental health sufferers. As with all public sector interventions, however, austerity has seen a decline in these services, impacting on availability and despite local initiatives, such as that taken by ASC with the MHTAs, are not bridging the enormity of reportedly increasing incidents. There is, of course, the moral dilemma too, that Sweeney (2015) points out in regard to the human right of choice and whether or not the extended arm of the law should reach beyond a person's decision to seek treatment.

In this chapter we have discussed some of the issues police officers face in the execution of their duty to those in crisis; restrictive legislation, a lack of training yet the expectation to 'fill the gap' of stripped-down mental health resources, ultimately leading to frustration of both officer and patient, with the person being kept in inappropriate surroundings without consultation or medical intervention for long periods of time. While there are some pockets of effective practice through the multi-agency approach used in triage services, the overarching summary is an 'out of depth' first-line of defence, where police officers try to manage situations and people without expertise or legislative support but who bear the burden of critique. The ultimate sacrifice, of course, are those who are in crisis, and their significant others who bear the brunt of crisis situations.

Further reading

- **Decriminalising mental illness:**

  Warburton, K. and Stahl, S.M. (eds) (2021) *Decriminalizing Mental Illness*. Cambridge: Cambridge University Press.
- **Mental health and crime:**

  Peay, J. (2017) Mental health, mental disabilities, and crime. In A. Leibling, S. Maruna and L. McAra (eds) *The Oxford Handbook of Criminology*, 6th edn. Oxford: Oxford University Press, pp. 639–662.
- **Police and people with mental illness:**

  Hacker, R.L. and Horan, J.J. (2019) Policing people with mental illness: Experimental evaluation of online training to de-escalate mental health crises. *Journal of Experimental Criminology*, 15, 551–567.
- **Twenty-first-century approach to mental health and policing:**

  Senior, J., Noga, H. and Shaw, J. (2014) When two worlds collide: A twenty-first century approach to mental health and policing. *Criminal Behaviour and Mental Health*, 24(2), 81–85.

References

Angiolini, E. (2017) *Report of the Independent Review of Deaths and Serious Incidents in Police Custody*. London: Home Office. Available at: https://www.gov.uk/government/publications/deaths-and-serious-incidents-in-police-custody (accessed 26 May 2021).

Care Act (2014) Section 44. Available at: https://www.legislation.gov.uk/ukpga/2014/23/section/44 (accessed 25 May 2021).

College of Policing (2016) Mental health APP. Available at: https://www.app.college.police.uk/app-content/mental-health/ (accessed 5 May 2021).

College of Policing (2018) Major investigation and public protection. Partnership working and multi-agency responses/mechanisms. Available at: https://www.app.college.police.uk/app-content/major-investigation-and-public-protection/domestic-abuse/partnership-working-and-multi-agency-responses/ (accessed 6 February 2021).

College of Policing (2020) Crisis Intervention Teams (CITs). Available at: https://what-works.college.police.uk/toolkit/Pages/Intervention (accessed 26 May 2021).

College of Policing (2021) Policing Education Qualifications Framework (PEQF). Available at: https://www.college.police.uk/career-learning/learning/PEQF (accessed 5 May 2021).

Criminal Justice and Courts Services Act 2000. S67 and S68. Available at: https://www.legislation.gov.uk/ukpga/2000/43/contents (accessed 13 April 2021).

Edwards, A. and Kotera, Y. (2020) Mental health in the UK police force: A qualitative investigation into the stigma with mental illness. *International Journal of Mental Health and Addiction*. Available at: https://link.springer.com/content/pdf/10.1007/s11469-019-00214-x.pdf (accessed 18 June).

Fox, J. (2019) The development of the police role in safeguarding children. In A. Pycroft and D. Gough (eds) *Multi-Agency Working in Criminal Justice: Theory, Policy and Practice*, 2nd edn. Bristol: Policy Press, pp. 121–138.

Gough, D. (2019) Multi-agency working and the governance of crime control. In A. Pycroft and D. Gough (eds) *Multi-Agency Working in Criminal Justice: Theory, Policy and Practice*, 2nd edn. Bristol: Policy Press, pp. 5–24.

HM Government and Mind (2014) Mental Health Crisis Care Concordat. Improving outcomes for people experiencing mental health crisis. Department of Health and Concordat signatories. Available at: https://assets.publishing.service.gov.uk/government/uploads/system/uploads/attachment_data/file/281242/36353_Mental_Health_Crisis_accessible.pdf (accessed 23 February 2021).

HMICFRS (Her Majesty's Inspectorate of Constabulary and Fire and Rescue Services) (2018a) Policing and Mental Health. Picking up the pieces. Available at: https://www.justiceinspectorates.gov.uk/hmicfrs/wp-content/uploads/policing-and-mental-health-picking-up-the-pieces.pdf (accessed 2 December 2020).

HMICFRS (Her Majesty's Inspectorate of Constabulary and Fire and Rescue Services) (2018b) What we do. Available at: https://www.justiceinspectorates.gov.uk/hmicfrs/about-us/what-we-do/ (accessed 25 May 2021).

Home Office (2019) *Police and Criminal Evidence Act 1984 Code C: Revised Code of Practice for the Detention, Treatment and Questioning of Persons by Police Officers.* Available at: https://www.gov.uk/government/publications/pace-code-c-2019 (accessed 25 May 2021).

Home Office (2020) *Crime and Police Statistics: Detentions under the Mental Health Act (1983)*. London: Home Office. Available at: https://assets.publishing.service.gov.uk/government/uploads/system/uploads/attachment_data/file/929091/detentions-mental-health-act-police-powers-procedures-mar20-tables.ods (accessed 26 May 2021).

Honess, R. (2020) Mandatory police training: The epitome of dissatisfaction and demotivation? *Policing*, 14(1), 191–201.

Jones, T., Newburn, R. and Reiner, R. (2017) Policing and the police. In A. Liebling, S. Maruna and L. McAra (eds) *The Oxford Handbook of Criminology*, 6th edn. Oxford: Oxford University Press, pp. 769–796.

Kane, E., Evans, E. and Shokraneh, F. (2017) Effectiveness of current policing-related mental health interventions in England and Wales and Crisis Intervention Teams as a future potential model: A systematic review. *Systematic Reviews*, 6(85), 1–7.

Kirubarajan, A., Puntis, S., Perfect, D., Tarbit, M., Buckman, M. and Molodynski, A. (2018) Street triage services in England: Service models, national provision and the opinions of police. *BJPsych Bulletin*, 42, 253–257.

Knauer, V., Walker, J. and Roberts, A. (2017) Offender personality disorder pathway: The impact of case consultation and formulation with probation staff. *The Journal of Forensic Psychiatry and Psychology*, 28(6), 825–840.

Leese, M. and Russell, S. (2017) Mental health, vulnerability and risk in police custody. *The Journal of Adult Protection*, 19(5), 274–283.

Lipsky, R. (1980) *Street Level Bureaucracy: Dilemmas of the Individual in Public Services*. New York: Russell Sage Foundation.

Loveday, B. and Roberts, S. (2019) A time of change: The expanding role of Police and Crime Commissioners in local criminal justice delivery. In A. Pycroft and D. Gough (eds) *Multi-Agency Working in Criminal Justice*, 2nd edn. Bristol: Policy Press, pp. 41–58.

Mental Capacity Act 2005. Available at: https://www.legislation.gov.uk/ukpga/2005/9/contents (accessed 1 June 2021).

Mental Capacity Act Codes of Practice 2007. Available at: https://www.gov.uk/government/publications/mental-capacity-act-code-of-practice (accessed 26 May 2021).

Mental Health Act 1983. Available at: https://www.legislation.gov.uk/ukpga/1983/20/contents (accessed 13 May 2021).

Mental Health Act 1983 Section 135. Available at: https://www.legislation.gov.uk/ukpga/1983/20/section/135 (accessed 25 May 2021).

Mental Health Act (1983) Section 136. Available at: https://www.legislation.gov.uk/ukpga/1983/20/section/136 (accessed 2 March 2021).

Mental Health First Aid (MHFD) (2020) *Mental Health Statistics*. Available at: https://mhfaengland.org/mhfa-centre/research-and-evaluation/mental-health-statistics/ (accessed 21 December 2020).

Ministry of Justice (2020) *Multi-Agency Public Protection Arrangements: Annual Report 2019/20*. Available at: https://assets.publishing.service.gov.uk/government/uploads/system/uploads/attachment_data/file/930302/MAPPA_Annual_Report_2019-20.pdf (accessed 28 February 2021).

Nash, M. (2010) The politics of public protection. In N. Nash and A. Williams (eds) *The Handbook of Public Protection*. Abingdon: Willan Publishing, pp. 60–62.

Office for National Statistics (2019) *Suicides in England and Wales: 2019 Registrations*. Available at: https://www.ons.gov.uk/peoplepopulationandcommunity/birthsdeathsandmarriages/deaths/bulletins/suicidesintheunitedkingdom/2019registrations (accessed 3 May 2021).

Oxford English Dictionary (2021) Arrest. Available at: https://www.oed.com (accessed 10 January 2021).

Pettitt, B., Koskela, S., Khalifeh, H., Drennan, V., Hart, T., Hogg, J., Borschmann, R., Mamo, E. and Moran, P. (2013). *At Risk Yet Dismissed: The Criminal Victimisation of People with Mental Health Problems*. Available at: https://www.researchgate.net/publication/264974122_At_risk_yet_dismissed_the_criminal_victimisation_of_people_with_mental_health_problems (accessed 25 May 2021).

Phillips, J., Padfield, N. and Gelsthorpe, L. (2018) Suicide and criminal justice. *Health and Justice*. Available at: https://healthandjusticejournal.biomedcentral.com/articles/10.1186/s40352-018-0072-7 (accessed 6 January 2021).

Pitts, J. (2018) Police reveal plan to stop people taking their own lives at Avon Gorge, *BristolLive*. Available at: https://www.bristolpost.co.uk/news/bristol-news/police-reveal-plan-stop-people-1743423 (accessed 1 January 2021).

Police and Criminal Evidence Act (1984) Section 24. Available at: https://www.legislation.gov.uk/ukpga/1984/60/section/24 (accessed 4 January 2021).

Police Federation (2018) The Office of Constable: The bedrock of modern-day British policing. Available at: https://www.polfed.org/media/14239/the-office-of-constable-with-links-2018 (accessed 11 June 2021).

Policing and Crime Act 2017. Available at: https://www.legislation.gov.uk/ukpga/2017/3/contents/enacted (accessed 13 May 2011).

Postans, A. (2019) Avon and Somerset police officers dealing with more than 100 mental health incidents a day. *Bristol Post*, 20 May 2020. Available at: https://www.bristolpost.co.uk/news/bristol-news/avon--somerset-police-officers-2885018 (accessed 5 January 2021).

Prison Reform Trust (2020) Mental health care in prisons. Available at: http://www.prisonreformtrust.org.uk/WhatWeDo/Projectsresearch/Mentalhealth (accessed 30 November 2020).

Rodgers, M., Thomas, S., Dalton, J., Harden, M. and Eastwood, A. (2019) Police-related triage interventions for mental health-related incidents: A rapid evidence synthesis. *Health Service and Delivery Research*, 7(20).

Sirdifield, C. and Brooker, C. (2020) Maximising positive mental health outcomes for people under probation supervision. Her Majesty's Inspectorate of Probation, Academic Insights 2020/06. Available at: https://www.justiceinspectorates.gov.uk/hmiprobation/wp-content/uploads/sites/5/2020/08/Maximising-positive-mental-health-outcomes-for-people-under-probation-supervision.pdf (accessed 21 December 2020).

Sweeney, F. (2015) Street triage – what, why and how, *The Psychologist*, 28, 676–677. Available at: https://thepsychologist.bps.org.uk/volume-28/august-2015/street-triage-what-why-and-how (accessed 25 May 2021).

Taheri, S.A. (2016) Do Crisis Intervention Teams reduce arrests and improve officer safety? A systematic review and meta-analysis. *Criminal Justice Police Review*, 27(1), 76–96.

Teplin, L.A. and Pruett, N.S. (1992) Police as streetcorner psychiatrist: Managing the mentally ill. *International Journal of Law and Psychiatry*, 15(2), 139–156.

Together for Mental Wellbeing (2020) Criminal Justice Services. Available at: https://www.together-uk.org/our-mental-health-services/criminal-justice-mental-health/ (accessed 21 December 2020).

UK Government (2021) Reforming the Mental Health Act: White Paper. Available at: https://assets.publishing.service.gov.uk/government/uploads/system/uploads/attachment_data/file/951398/mental-health-act-white-paper-web-accessible.pdf (accessed 5 May 2021).

Warrington, C. (2019) Repeated Police Mental Health Act detentions in England and Wales: Trauma and recurrent suicidality. *International Journal of Environmental Research and Public Health*, 16, 4786. Available at: https://doi.org/10.3390/ijerph16234786.

Winstone, J. (2019) Offenders with mental health needs in the criminal justice system: The multi-agency challenge to provide solution-focused response. In A. Pycroft and D. Gough (eds) *Multi-agency Working in Criminal Justice*, 2nd edn. Bristol: Policy Press, pp. 237–254.

Wondemaghen, M. (2021) Policing mental illness: Police use of Section 136 – Perspectives from police and mental-health nurses. *Medicine, Science, and the Law*. Available at: https://doi.org/10.1177/0025802421993363.

5   The role of the paramedic in mental health crisis care

David Williams

The chapter will explore the relationship between paramedics working in a frontline ambulance role and individuals experiencing a mental health crisis. The aim is to provide an outline of the paramedic role for other professionals but also to act as a resource to paramedics who may be looking to develop their own knowledge around mental healthcare. The first section of the chapter will discuss the contemporary paramedic role and identify the scope of practice and professional obligations in relation to mental healthcare. Thereafter, some key concepts and challenges faced by the paramedic clinician will be explored when attending mental health-related incidents, including risk assessment and appropriate referral pathways. The chapter will then discuss the importance of shared decision making and collaborative working while providing emergency mental healthcare, also with consideration of the paramedic interaction with other professional groups. Finally, the chapter will delve into the concept of good working practice; this will explore best practice not only from a clinical care perspective but also from an organisational standpoint with recommendations for change.

Introduction

Unlike many of the other professions reflected within this book, the paramedic profession is very much in its infancy. Not that the profession lacks some form of professional attributes yet to be developed, but in recognition of the rapid professionalisation and development of the role of the paramedic over the last 50 years. Historically, the role of the 'ambulance driver' has been simply to transport patients to hospital rapidly, providing minimal intervention that could affect patient outcomes (Newton, 2012). This position began to change in the late twentieth century with the established role of the 'extended trained ambulance staff' programme from the Department of Health (DH) and subsequent professional registration of paramedics (College of Paramedics, 2020a). More recent developments include the education threshold for paramedic registration to be raised to a minimum of a level 6 degree – indicating graduation from higher education – and diversification away from roles within the ambulance service (Eaton *et al.*, 2020; Health and Care Professions Council, 2018).

It is of note that the chapter will focus on the role of frontline paramedics within an ambulance service role. Paramedics working within other clinical settings would be expected to provide clinical care akin to their nursing and medical colleagues. For example, paramedics working within the emergency department (ED) setting would provide a similar assessment, management and referral of patients experiencing a mental health crisis to that outlined in Chapter 2. Similarly, a 999-ambulance response will not always have a paramedic clinician on board and there are a range of other clinical roles such as emergency care assistants, ambulance technicians and ambulance nurses who may respond in an ambulance vehicle. These roles vary significantly across the country, but much of the information in this chapter will be applicable to these other roles in terms of structure, general approach and considerations. Nevertheless, the paramedic, as discussed in this chapter, is interpreted in terms of a frontline paramedic ambulance service role.

It is important when discussing paramedic care of mental health crisis to understand the prevalence of this condition. However, it is challenging to find accurate statistical data to identify the scale of the presentation of mental health crisis to the ambulance service. This is partly due to the range of undifferentiated information received initially from a 999 call. For example, the call reporting an individual is suffering from breathing difficulties could subsequently turn out to be hyperventilation secondary to a mental health crisis. Similarly, there are issues with identifying data from diagnostic coding at the end of a clinical encounter. The individual suffering a mental health crisis who has self-harmed may receive a primary diagnosis code on the clinical records system related to their wound (e.g. 'laceration').

Despite challenges with accurate data recording, one recent article explored mental health-related callouts within the Scottish Ambulance Service (Duncan *et al.*, 2019), finding that mental health-related calls accounted for 11 per cent of the overall call volume. Importantly, the article identifies as the first UK research exploring ambulance callouts and clinical outcomes in mental health-related emergencies and suggests, 'both the ambulance service and Emergency Departments are currently missing opportunities to provide better care to this vulnerable population. This results in potentially avoidable mortality, increased levels of patient morbidity, and service burden' (Duncan *et al.*, 2019, p. 7). This article will be explored again later, but its stark recommendations provide the important context within this introduction.

The figure of 11 per cent may initially be perceived as relatively small, however, it is important that the figure is contextualised. For example, data suggests that only 9 per cent of ambulance callouts related to 'category 1' emergencies are calls deemed to be life-threatening conditions, such as cardiac arrest (Nuffield Trust, 2020). Therefore, mental health-related calls make up a greater percentage of callouts, opposing views perhaps held by the public and other professionals associated with the traditional paramedic role. Despite frequent exposure to mental health-related incidents, paramedic confidence with related assessment and management is low. Rolfe, Pope and Crouch (2020, p. 1) found paramedics felt 'frustrated and unsupported when dealing with patients experiencing mental health issues' and, similarly, a survey of paramedics by Berry (2014) identified virtually unanimous recommendations for further training in managing mental health calls.

Concern among paramedics in terms of their competence and confidence in mental healthcare is undoubtedly multifaceted, including education, shared decision making and identifying appropriate treatment pathways; all of which will be explored further. However, also important is acknowledging the perception of attending mental health-related callouts among paramedics. The article by Rolfe, Pope and Crouch (2020) suggests that a number of participants felt mental health-related calls were not 'emergencies'. Notably,

> Many paramedics felt that responding to calls requiring assistance for a mental health problem was not part of the emergency work they had been trained to do. Their ideal role was to respond to life threatening emergencies, and patients experiencing mental health issues were not always considered an emergency.

While such mentality reflects a lack of training in mental healthcare, there is need to explore guidance mandating paramedic care in supporting individuals experiencing a mental health crisis.

The Mental Health Crisis Care Concordat, published in 2014, is a 'national agreement between services and agencies involved in the care and support of people in crisis' (HM Government and Mind, 2014). The concordat outlines the need to recognise a mental health crisis as a health emergency and suggests the role the ambulance service should adopt within community crisis care. Notably the concordat adopts a multi-professional perspective recognising the role paramedics can provide in complementing the skills of their policing, mental health, and ED colleagues among others. Additionally, the paramedic focus on good mental healthcare is another key consideration of parity of esteem. The government strategy, drawn up in 2011, sets out the integral need to prioritise mental health equally alongside physical healthcare (HM Government, 2011). Perhaps most importantly from the paramedic perspective, the agenda also recognises that there is a false dichotomy between mental and physical health and, realistically, many people suffer with a combination of mental and physical illness. Therefore, it could be concluded that for a paramedic to provide effective urgent and emergency care, they must be skilled, confident, and willing to manage both an individual's physical and mental health needs.

Defining crisis and appropriate paramedic response

The introduction to the chapter explored the role of the paramedic, the frequent exposure paramedics have to mental health-related calls and the importance of the paramedic being supported to provide both effective mental and physical healthcare in the community. However, also significant is understanding the definition and presentation of 'mental health crisis' within the paramedic context. As alluded to elsewhere in this book, mental health crisis is a subjective term when an individual may feel that their mental health is at 'breaking point' (Mind, 2020). Paramedics, by the nature of responding to undifferentiated emergencies via the 999 system, are likely to respond to a crisis scenario when attending mental health-related callouts. For clarity, some examples of common mental health-related callouts for paramedic and other ambulance staff are detailed below:

- An individual has taken an overdose and has contacted their mental health support worker. The support worker has advised them to call 999 for an ambulance.
- An individual is experiencing suicidal ideation and has taken themselves to a public place (e.g. a bridge). A member of the public has become concerned and called 999 for the police and ambulance service.
- An individual is experiencing a mental health crisis and is having thoughts of self-harm. Family and friends have received communication from the individual and have become concerned. They have called 111 for advice and an emergency ambulance has been deemed the appropriate response.

The purpose of the examples is to outline some types of mental health crises attended by paramedics, but also to help readers place themselves in the mindset of the paramedic. The above information would be akin to what paramedics may receive on the way to an incident while responding on blue lights and sirens. It is unlikely that the paramedic will have any prior knowledge of the individual, while it is also unusual for paramedics to access the individual's digital health record, such as a mental health crisis plan, although accessibility to records is gradually improving (Hughes, 2019; NHS Digital, 2019). The lack of information that paramedics may face is challenging but would be similar to other non-mental health-related incidents. Therefore, the primary task for a paramedic attending a mental health crisis is to obtain a history, including a clinical history, but also considerations specific to community care including the location and setting of the clinical encounter. For example, if called to a crowded public place, the paramedic will need to consider the best strategy to maintain the patient's privacy and dignity, which may involve encouraging the patient into the back of the ambulance. However, at the same time, the paramedic must be aware of the safety and risk to themselves and colleagues in the confines of such a space.

Before exploring further concepts and options available to paramedics to help support individuals experiencing crisis, within the context of the ambulance service, recognition is needed that a 999 call does not necessarily mean a face-to-face assessment (i.e. an ambulance attends the scene of the incident). 'Hear and treat' is the term attached to 999 calls managed without the dispatch of an ambulance vehicle (Bishop-Edwards *et al.*, 2017). Hear and treat is undertaken by a range of clinicians including paramedics, nurses, doctors and mental health specialists. Data from April 2021 suggests that of all calls received by the ambulance service, 8.4 per cent were managed via hear and treat (NHS England, 2021). The importance of developing safe hear and treat processes within ambulance services is uncontested, in that the number of available ambulances to respond to calls is a finite resource. Moreover, ambulances need to be available to rapidly respond to life-threatening category 1 calls, as previously outlined. However, in consideration of mental health crisis, ambulance services using hear and treat need to ensure appropriate onward referral and information sharing to mental health teams to provide safe ongoing care. Exploring paramedic perspectives of managing mental health crisis via hear and treat, Briggs, Clarke and Rees (2021) found a low level of confidence and inadequacies in the referral pathways available. Hence, further research exploring patient experiences of ambulance hear and treat in relation to mental health crisis would be of value to develop this intervention.

Risk assessment

Within the patient interaction, after obtaining a history and assessing the scene, the paramedic would then conduct a physical and mental health assessment. Earlier, the interaction between physical and mental health was touched upon, and it is important to recognise the role that a physical health assessment, such as clinical observations, plays in helping to identify the most appropriate care for individuals, even when the cause is believed to be a mental health crisis.

Consider the example of a person presenting to the paramedic in an acutely distressed state, the individual is alone in a public place and obtaining a history of events is challenging. When the paramedic undertakes a physical health assessment, they identify significant symptoms like tachycardia, tachypnoea and hypoxia (rapid heart rate, rapid breathing and lack of oxygen respectively). These would very much dictate that the ED is the most appropriate place for this individual. While a simplified example, it could also become apparent from the same initial information that the paramedic suspects a mental health crisis, and a physical health assessment can provide reassurance that urgent physical care is not needed. Anecdotally, differentiating between a primary physical or mental illness in the pre-hospital setting is challenging and paramedics play a key role in being competent and well equipped to undertake physical health assessments. Also significant is that it can be impossible in the pre-hospital setting to differentiate between mental and physical illness, and, as suggested, the individual may in fact be presenting with a combination of the two.

In terms of mental health assessment, many tenets of a robust acute mental health assessment are well outlined in Chapter 2. However, there are unique considerations faced by paramedics, particularly with regards to risk assessment in relation to patients expressing suicidal ideation. Paramedics have access to a range of clinical guidance designed to support their assessment and management of patients. These include the Joint Royal Colleges Ambulance

Liaison Committee (JRCALC) guidance which provides information on a vast array of clinical topics (JRCALC, 2021). One such guideline is titled 'Mental Health Presentation: Crisis, Distress and Disordered Behaviour' and is aimed at supporting ambulance clinicians in managing mental health-related calls (JRCALC and Association of Ambulance Chief Executives (AACE), 2019, p. 289). This guidance recommends the use of the IPAP Suicide Risk Assessment Tool, which it suggests is 'a basic suicide risk assessment process that can be used by non-mental health professionals to identify and assess the presence of a suicide risk'. IPAP stands for 'Intent, Plan, Action and Protective measures' (JRCALC and AACE, 2019).

The challenge faced by the paramedic having navigated through the questions of the IPAP tool is what to do with this information. When IPAP was first introduced into the JRCALC guidance, a risk-level matrix was provided to help paramedics interpret the information obtained within the IPAP tool. However, this risk matrix was subsequently removed for contravening guidance from the National Institute for Clinical Excellence (NICE). NICE advised against using risk assessment tools and scales due to their inaccuracy at predicting risk of suicide (AACE, 2021; NICE, 2011). Nevertheless, NICE support the use of an assessment tool such as IPAP, if it provides structure to a risk assessment and includes the questions from their recommended list. To access these questions, a link can be found in the further reading section concluding the chapter (NICE, 2011).

While it is useful that national guidance aligns with ambulance service clinical guidance, it could be argued that a lacuna is left for the paramedic, who previously relied on this risk matrix to help formulate a clinical plan. Therefore, in the absence of an evidence-based pre-hospital suicide risk assessment scale, the paramedic should consider the following points in ensuring good risk assessment. First, have a low threshold to liaise with other agencies, for example, the Crisis Resolution and Home Treatment Team (CRHTT) to discuss previous risk assessments and a crisis plan, if available, as this may provide useful information unobtainable at the scene of the incident. Second, carefully consider the support network the patient may have, particularly when considering discharging the patient on the scene. Finally, ensure there is a good awareness of risk factors in relation to suicide. In a similar vein to physical illness such as cardiovascular disease, understanding the risk factors or 'red flags' for suicide can help to support decision making (RCP, 2020, p. 37). However, as with cardiovascular disease, a myocardial infarction can occur without any risk factors; hence, in the absence of suicide risk factors, the risk is not necessarily eliminated, and the risk assessment process should be specific to that individual.

Navigating the legal framework

Consider the example that once the paramedic has undertaken their history-taking, physical and mental health assessment, they consider the individual to be at substantial risk of suicide. The paramedic believes in their professional judgement, that if they leave this individual, there is a high chance of imminent harm. However, the individual is adamantly refusing to receive further support with their mental health. To understand ways forward from such a scenario, this section will explore the various legal mechanisms available to support the provision of safe and appropriate care for the individual.

Section 136 of the Mental Health Act (1983)

While policing colleagues in Chapter 4 have discussed their perspective of the role of Section 136 of the Mental Health Act (MHA, 1983), it is important to understand the paramedic considerations of this legal power of detention. Amendments to Section 136 of the MHA were brought in under the Policing and Crime Act 2017. These provisions included a duty on the police constable to consult a healthcare professional when practicable prior to deciding to implement Section 136. While paramedics are not specifically listed within the legislation, it is common to be asked by a police officer for a paramedic opinion on the use of Section 136. Although recognising that many paramedics are not mental health experts, it is important to consider some of the issues associated with the use of Section 136.

First, in regard to Section 136, there is consideration around the experience of the individual. Sondhi *et al.* (2018) undertook research exploring patient perspectives of being detained under Section 136. Interestingly, concern among participants focused less on a principled concern with emergency mental health detention powers but more around process and the patient-professional relationship. One participant stated, 'It was all too long in the back of an ambulance, and no one gave me any information as to what was going on … I became paranoid that I was being abducted' (Sondhi *et al.*, 2018, p. 162). While the Crisis Care Concordat (HM Government and Mind, 2014) mandates the use of ambulances rather than police vehicles for Section 136 conveyance, this quote demonstrates the value that a paramedic can bring in supporting an individual who has been detained under Section 136, particularly with providing reassurance and communication about the processes involved.

Second, it is important to consider the necessity of Section 136. The legislation states Section 136 should be applied when the police constable believes the individual 'to be in immediate need of care or control' (MHA, 1983). This term 'immediate' may be queried by the police constable with paramedics on the scene. Therefore, it is an important consideration for the paramedic whether the individual will voluntarily be conveyed for further assessment and support, as it may then raise questions if a mandatory detention is required in the first place. Paramedics will also need to ensure that a thorough health check occurs in case an emergency department is required, as explored in case study 5.1.

Case study 5.1 Paramedics and Section 136 process

An ambulance has been requested by police officers who have detained an individual under Section 136 at a local train station.

On arrival, the paramedic-led crew find the individual in a highly distressed state. Alongside undertaking a physical health assessment, the ambulance crew are able to develop a rapport with the individual, using the back of the ambulance to provide a calm environment. Based on the paramedic assessment, it is deemed that a place of safety suite is an appropriate destination for the patient and no interventions are needed within the emergency department. The paramedic collaborates with the police officer to discuss the individual's care with the place of safety suite team.

MCA versus MHA

Despite Section 136 having a significant role in supporting individuals in need of immediate assessment, it cannot be applied in an individual's own home. Therefore, given the example at the start of this discussion around the law and now considering the individual is in their own home, in terms of legal frameworks, the paramedic has two key options to consider: the Mental Capacity Act (MCA, 2005) and other provisions within the MHA. While it is beyond the scope of the chapter to discuss in detail the application of the MCA, it is covered further in Chapters 2 and 6. Nevertheless, in summary, where an individual is felt to lack mental capacity in relation to a specific decision, a decision must be made in their best interests, which may include appropriate and proportionate restraint to facilitate treatment or transport.

For the paramedic, the apparent challenge with selecting the MCA or MHA (with support from other professionals, i.e. Approved Mental Health Professionals (AMHP)) is the most appropriate option in a given situation. Some clarity can be found, as discussed in Chapter 4 on the police, by exploring case law. *R (Sessay) v South London and Maudsley NHS Foundation Trust and The Commissioner of Police for the Metropolis* [2011] EWHC 2617 (QB) was a case when police officers used the powers within Section 5 of the MCA to convey an individual suffering a mental health crisis to a place of safety. However, this was ruled unlawful, and the powers contained within the MHA should have been applied, specifically Section 4 – emergency detainment of up to 72 hours for the purpose of assessment (MHA, 1983) – in conjunction with an AMHP. Principally this makes sense, although challenges exist in accessing the support of a mental health professional at any time of day, discussed later on in the chapter.

The MCA may still play a role in an incident related to a mental health crisis. For example, consider a patient who has taken a large overdose and is in a semi-conscious state on the arrival of the paramedics. In this situation, a mental health crisis highlights a physical health emergency. Accordingly, the MCA may be used to formulate a best interests decision, likely leading to conveyance of that individual to the ED under the provisions of Section 5 of the MCA. Interestingly, concern was raised in the aforementioned *Sessay v SLAM* case for the lack of scope for the MCA to allow the deprivation of an individual's liberty. However, Department of Health (DH, 2015) guidance would suggest that an ambulance conveyance would very rarely contribute to a deprivation of liberty and instead be recognised as a temporary restriction of liberty. The interface between the MCA and MHA can lead to confusion among professionals and an argument has been made for developing a combined piece of law covering the realms of both the MCA and the MHA, a so-called 'fusion law' (Dawson and Szmukler, 2006). In the absence of a fusion law, the challenging interface between the MCA and the MHA needs to be successfully navigated by the paramedic. As such, the emphasis on accessing senior decision-making support when navigating the interface between the MCA and MHA cannot be understated (Bartlett, 2019).

Conveyance or discharge

Once the paramedic has undertaken an assessment and considered whether there is a need to use either the MHA or MCA, they will then decide on conveyance. In some situations, such as an individual placed under Section 136 by a police constable, the paramedic will help to facilitate safe transport to a place of safety, a location often arranged by the police constable in line with local agreements. In other mental health crisis situations, the paramedic will need to decide whether conveyance to the ED, referral to a mental health service or discharge on scene is appropriate. This is specific to a range of factors in a given situation, but this section of the chapter will highlight some concerns around the ED for individuals in crisis while recognising there is often a lack of suitable alternatives. It will also outline the standards expected when a paramedic discharges an individual at the scene of an incident including producing a 'safety netting' plan.

The emergency department

Paramedics spend a considerable proportion of their working lives in the ED, conveying patients for an array of conditions. Although it is worth recognising that of all the emergency calls attended by paramedics, approximately 30 per cent are managed on scene without conveyance to hospital (NHS England, 2021). The figure is somewhat lower for mental health-related calls at approximately 11 per cent (Duncan *et al.*, 2019). This suggests many individuals experiencing a mental health crisis are conveyed to the ED, while the recommendation that 'patients in mental health crisis ideally should be conveyed to 24/7 mental health referral assessment units', is simply not an available option in most of the country (NHS England, 2015, p. 11). The challenge arises in the ability of the ED to provide a 'safe, therapeutic environment' for these patients (CQC, 2020). This is reflected by some difficult experiences of EDs by patients when suffering a mental health crisis (Thomas *et al.*, 2019).

There are many situations when paramedics attend to mental health difficulties when the ED is the most appropriate option. For example, a patient requiring wound closure or intoxication, meaning they are unsafe to remain on scene but cannot undergo a mental health assessment (RCP, 2020). Equally, situations exist when individuals are conveyed to the ED who could have been safely and effectively managed in the community. While there appears little literature exploring exactly when it is appropriate to discharge a person experiencing a mental health crisis in the community, it is important when considering conveyance to ED, questions are raised about whether other options are available. Indeed, community care does not equal no care, hence discharge should conclude with safe and effective referrals, most likely to a mental health team.

Discharge and safety netting

In situations when paramedics are discharging individuals who have called the ambulance service following a mental health crisis in the community, as well as discussing or referring the details of the call to the mental health team, they should formulate a safety plan with the patient. The phrase 'safety netting' is commonly used in paramedic practice. However, how safety netting advice is used in clinical practice varies between clinicians (O'Hara *et al.*, 2015). Alternatively, the phrase 'safety plan' may be used in the context of mental health crisis care, as per guidance from the Royal College of Psychiatrists (RCP, 2020, p. 49). In reality, safety netting and safety plan reflect similar ideas. The ambulance services should equip paramedics with the ability to formulate safety plans with patients who have called 999 for mental health difficulties who are discharged on the scene. This plan should include, but not be limited to, contact information in case the situation worsens, distraction activities, reduced access to lethal means of suicide and strategies to help manage further worsening of the crisis episode, including the support of social networks (i.e. friends and family) (RCP, 2020). Anecdotally, a safety plan pro-forma for mental health crisis care is currently not commonplace within the ambulance service setting. However, ambulance services should consider adopting this principle into clinical guidance to reduce risk of future mortality and morbidity in patients at risk of self-harm or suicide (Duncan *et al.*, 2019).

Collaboration with stakeholders

Given that the guiding principle of this book is one of collaboration, paramedics will interact with a vast range of professionals and service users during their professional lives. Frequent interactions with police and ED colleagues have already been highlighted. However, the focus within this section will discuss the patient, friends, family, and mental health teams alongside their interaction with paramedics.

The patient

So far, the terms patient, individual and service user have been used to describe a person who may be experiencing a mental health crisis. While they have been used synonymously, they of course carry a social meaning which is important for the paramedic to consider when providing care. Indeed, that is the key consideration within this passage, that over-medicalisation and paternalism in the management of mental health crisis are problematic. Paternalism in healthcare stems from the idea that 'the doctor knows best' and that treatment decisions have been traditionally made by clinicians without patient input (Jackson, 2018). However, with regard to mental healthcare, it is important to promote individual autonomy and for the paramedic to adopt a stance of patient-centred decision making (Breeze, 2001; Carver, Moritz and Ebbs, 2020; Pelto-Piri, Engstrom and Engstrom; 2013). Practically, this involves making sure the individual's voice is heard within the decision-making process. The challenge, as Breeze (2001) suggests, is around the interaction between patient-centred decision making and a paternalistic legal framework (e.g. mandatory detention for mental illness against individual wishes). Nevertheless, even in cases where the MHA is being sought for mandatory detention by the paramedic with the assistance of other helping professionals, interpreting and considering the patient's viewpoint within this interaction are still of significant importance.

Friends and family

Friends, family and others present at the scene of a 999 call are an important consideration for the paramedic. It is common for paramedics to attend traumatic scenes, for example, in the context of deliberate self-harm. While paramedic clinicians may have a range of support available for their own mental well-being, the well-being of friends and family who have witnessed events and called for the ambulance needs to be considered. This may include options such as signposting individuals to seek support from primary care services or towards the directory of services to support their mental health such as Hub of Hope (2021). Hub of Hope is a database of mental health support and is a useful tool to help navigate the range of different support services that are available locally.

Another consideration regarding friends and family for the paramedic is their ability to support an individual experiencing a mental health crisis. There is a significant role for the paramedic to liaise with and consider the viewpoints of significant others, with the consent of the patient, when attending a mental health crisis (Javed and Herrman, 2017). Such collaboration not only provides reassurance in terms of available support when discharging patients on scene, but also helps to promote patient autonomy by understanding what the individual may want, involving their mental healthcare. This is particularly beneficial when it is challenging to interpret the views of the patient in conditions such as psychosis.

Collaborating with mental health teams

When attending mental health-related callouts in the community, it was suggested that the paramedic should have a low threshold to engage with mental health teams such as CRHTT. Benefits of engagement can be numerous, and include if information is available, gaining a greater understanding of the patient's history alongside assessments such as involving risk. Shared decision making with a mental health professional is important to ensure an appropriate and safe clinical plan is implemented, while information sharing can aid the continuity of mental healthcare. Nonetheless, access for paramedics to mental health crisis teams varies and is particularly challenging in the context of children and young people (Lloyd-Evans *et al.*, 2018; Prothero and Cooke, 2016). Issues are exacerbated by the 24/7 nature of ambulance responses and lack of other clinical decision support mechanisms, notably the unavailability of the patient's own GP, contactable only during daytime hours. Therefore, ambulance services should work with commissioning groups to ensure 24/7 access for paramedics to mental health clinicians to support on-scene decision-making (NHS England, 2018).

Interactions with services like the CRHTT can be challenging for the paramedic, and lead to frustration, particularly when services have different interpretation of the appropriate action in each situation (Rolfe, Pope and Crouch, 2020). To increase the positive interaction between paramedics and mental health clinicians, both professional groups have an obligation to educate themselves on the other's approach to care. For paramedic colleagues, Chapter 3 of this book may prove a useful starting point, alongside identifying collaborative training opportunities with local mental health professionals. Similarly, for mental health colleagues, it is important to understand the approaches adopted by paramedics as outlined in this chapter, while the further reading section may prove useful to develop an understanding of paramedic practice.

Good practice and recommendations

Earlier sections of the chapter outlined how paramedics have a key role in mental health crisis care and have frequent clinical exposure to this presentation. However, it has also been explained that paramedic confidence in assessing and managing mental health crisis is low (Berry, 2014; Rolfe, Pope and Crouch, 2020). Similarly, Duncan *et al.* (2019) explored mortality and morbidity associated with ambulance service callouts to mental health emergencies. It was suggested that 'the ambulance service therefore have a unique opportunity to deliver a range of potential suicide prevention strategies through developing alternative care pathways to specialist mental health services, delivering suicide prevention interventions' (Duncan *et al.*, 2019, p. 6). The aim of this concluding section is to outline good practice, including case studies analysing the effect of these interventions. This will be considered in three different domains related to paramedic practice: (1) multi-agency response; (2) education; and (3) specialist practice.

Multi-agency response

Multi-agency response in relation to ambulance service callouts for mental healthcare is not a new phenomenon. In 2014, Birmingham and Solihull Mental Health NHS Foundation Trust teamed up with the West Midlands Ambulance Service and West Midlands Police to provide a joint response in a 'street triage car' to mental health-related 999 calls (BSMHFT, 2015). The team consists of a mental health nurse, a paramedic, and a police officer. They suggest that each of these professional groups brings a unique skillset to provide improved outcomes and quality in care. They also provide impressive statistics of their impact. 'In the first year of its operation there was a 50% reduction in Section 136 detainments due to the positive interventions of the team at the scene of a crisis' (BSMHFT, 2015). A more recent pilot evaluation of a similar scheme in London with a band 7 mental health nurse and a paramedic also provides convincing data to its effectiveness, markedly an 80.7 per cent 'see and treat' rate versus 45.6 per cent 'see and treat' for 'business as usual' responses (NHS England and NHS Improvement, 2020). This report also outlines improved patient satisfaction and reduced cost burden to the overall health system, with no identified increase in clinical risk. However, despite the potential benefit of these multi-agency crisis teams, such services are not widely available 24/7 across the UK (Cook, 2019). Whenever possible, as explored in the concluding chapter, local initiatives should be implemented for ambulance services to work collaboratively with local commissioning groups and partner mental health trusts, to fine-tune integrated systems and improve the cohesion of mental health crisis care.

Education

A consistent theme within the literature surrounding the feelings paramedics have when responding to mental health crisis is a lack of education and training about the subject (Berry, 2014; Rees *et al.*, 2018; Rolfe, Pope and Crouch, 2020). This sentiment reflects the study findings exploring evidence-based approaches to paramedic education, suggesting the 'development of ... mental health awareness knowledge and skills is a priority for the students and the qualified paramedic workforce. Much of the knowledge in this field is gained through observation' (Lovegrove and Davis, 2013, p. 77). However, questions arise with deciding exactly what level of mental health knowledge, assessment and management skills paramedics should receive at a pre- and post-registration level. Profession-specific curriculum guidance appears vague, merely emphasising the importance of covering mental healthcare as part of paramedic education (College of Paramedics, 2019).

The points raised about education are significant. A review of paramedic mental health education in Australia found considerable variations between different paramedic degree programmes and the level of education provided (Smith *et al.*, 2020). This is while a UK study of one education programme suggests that students are not properly equipped to assess and manage the needs of those requiring mental healthcare (Hutchison *et al.*, 2019). While variations between local health systems may exist, these should not deter developing a consistent and evidence-based approach to mental health education on UK paramedic training programmes. Education should include, but not be limited to, the approaches outlined in this chapter, notably mental health assessment, risk assessment, shared decision making and patient-centred care. Similarly, post-registration training could be advanced by multi-disciplinary education modules to build collaborative approaches between mental health clinicians, paramedics and other professionals. Through sharing awareness and knowledge, these modules might provide fertile ground to develop local integrative systems with a view to promote interprofessional mental healthcare.

Specialist practice

The benefits of a multi-agency response to ambulance service calls for mental health crisis have been outlined, including providing a mental health specialist such as a mental health nurse to attend these incidents. However, another option is to introduce and develop a mental health specialism within the paramedic domain (Cook, 2019). As suggested, paramedics are diversifying and specialising in a range of roles away from traditional emergency ambulance practice, including among others, primary care and critical care (College of Paramedics, 2020b). However, the role of the 'specialist paramedic in mental healthcare' is not commonplace. The benefits of developing mental health expertise and specialism within the paramedic profession are potentially numerous. These include shared education among paramedic and ambulance colleagues improving confidence in mental health practice, the patient benefit of a timely and consistent 24/7 response to community mental health crisis, and perhaps, economic benefits in comparison to systems using a paramedic and a mental health nurse. In addition, paramedic-specific focus on mental healthcare may enable the implementation of system improvements, such as the recommendation of the use of bespoke crisis vehicles in the Wessely Review (Department of Health and Social Care, 2018).

The development of paramedic mental health specialist practice may also lead to recognition that emergency detention powers for mental health-related emergencies sit more appropriately within the domain of the paramedic rather than police constable. Other jurisdictions such as Australia have adopted this approach, prioritising police involvement where there are safety concerns (Bradbury, Ireland and Stasa, 2014). However, any movement to extending or shifting legal powers towards the paramedic profession must be accompanied by examining the impact on the patient-paramedic relationship and careful governance to avoid unnecessary legal detention for mental illness (Bradley, Townsend and Eburn, 2015; Keown *et al.*, 2016). Irrespective of whether there is a need to direct legislation to paramedic practice, due to the regular exposure of the ambulance service to mental health crisis, a cost-benefit analysis and pilot study of the 'mental health specialist paramedic' would be valuable, to identify the potential impact of this novel role.

Conclusion

The paramedic profession plays a unique but vital role in the care of individuals experiencing a mental health crisis. Despite frequent exposure to mental health-related incidents, paramedic confidence in assessing and managing mental illness is low. Additionally, there are significant and repeated calls from the paramedic profession and wider policy to develop evidence-based approaches to mental health education for the paramedic at both a pre- and post-registration level. Nevertheless, despite these challenges, paramedics bring a combination of physical and mental health assessment skills to the undifferentiated emergency incident. As such, ambulance services should continue to improve tools that support safe and effective care, including safety planning documentation.

Furthermore, the data suggests there is scope and opportunity to innovate the ambulance service response to mental health calls to improve patient satisfaction and reduce mortality and morbidity. Initiatives such as the street triage car and the London joint response car pilot demonstrate impressive statistics to justify their implementation nationally. Additionally, the potential for the development of a new role of a 'mental health specialist paramedic' represents an exciting opportunity for the profession and wider stakeholders, to ensure mental health-related incidents truly are treated with parity of esteem.

Further reading

- **London mental health joint response car pilot review:**
  NHSI and London Ambulance Service (2020) NHS England and NHS Improvement. Mental Health Joint Response Car Pilot – Evaluation Report. Available at: https://aace.org.uk/wp-content/uploads/2020/08/MHJRC-Review-Final-12082020.pdf (accessed 14 April 2021).
- **Mental health law, ethics and paramedic care:**
  Eaton, G. (2019) *Law and Ethics for Paramedics: An Essential Guide.* Bridgwater: Class Professional Publishing.
- **NICE guidance including recommended points to consider when undertaking a risk assessment:**

NICE (2011) *Self-harm in Over 8s: Long-Term Management*. Available at: https://www.nice.org.uk/guidance/cg133/chapter/1-Guidance (accessed 2 May 2021).

• **Paramedic guidance of mental health crisis:**

JRCALC and AACE (2019) *JRCALC Clinical Guideline: National Ambulance Service Clinical Guidance for the Management of Mental Health Related Incidents*. Bridgwater: Class Professional Publishing.

References

AACE (2021) *Mental Health Presentation: Removal of Risk Levels*. Available at: https://aace.org.uk/jrcalc-updates-2019/mental-health-presentation-removal-of-risk-levels/ (accessed 2 May 2021).

Bartlett, E. (2019) Assessing mental capacity. In G. Eaton (ed.) *Law and Ethics for Paramedics*. Bridgwater: Class Professional Publishing.

Berry, M. (2014) College of Paramedics evidence into mental health care and policing. *Journal of Paramedic Practice*, 6(10), 539–540.

Bishop-Edwards, L., Knowles, E., Ahmed, N. and O'Cathain, A. (2017) Exploring 'hear and treat' practices in three ambulance service trusts. *Emergency Medicine Journal*. Available at: https://emj.bmj.com/content/34/10/e10.2 (accessed 22 April 2021).

Bradbury, J., Ireland, M. and Stasa, H. (2014) Mental health emergency transport: The pot-holed road to care. *The Medical Journal of Australia*, 199, 288–292.

Bradley, E.J., Townsend, R. and Eburn, M. (2015) Paramedics and ACT mental health legislation. *Australasian Journal of Paramedicine*, 12(4), 1–6.

Breeze, J. (2001) Can paternalism be justified in mental health care? *Journal of Advanced Nursing*, 28(2), 260–265.

Briggs, H., Clarke, S. and Rees, N. (2021) Mental health assessment and triage in an ambulance clinical contact centre. *Journal of Paramedic Practice*, 13(5), 196–203.

BSMHFT (2015) *Street Triage*. Available at: https://www.bsmhft.nhs.uk/our-services/urgent-care/street-triage/#:~:text=A%20Street%20Triage%20car%20will,a%20plain%20ambulance%20response%20vehicle (accessed 15 May 2021).

Carver, H., Moritz, D. and Ebbs, P. (2020) Ethics and law in paramedic practice: Boundaries of capacity and interests. *Journal of Paramedic Practice*, 12(10), 1–8.

College of Paramedics (2019) *Paramedic Curriculum Guidance*, 5th edn. Available at: https://collegeofparamedics.co.uk/COP/ProfessionalDevelopment/Paramedic_Curriculum_Guidance.aspx (accessed 1 May 2021).

College of Paramedics (2020a) *The Journey of the College of Paramedics*. Available at: https://collegeofparamedics.co.uk/COP/About_Us/The_Journey_of_the_College.aspx (accessed 23 March 2021).

College of Paramedics (2020b) *Interactive Career Framework*. Available at: https://www.collegeofparamedics.co.uk/COP/Professional_development/interactive_career_framework/COP/ProfessionalDevelopment/Interactive_Career_Framework.aspx?hkey=5058228a-13ef-4d38-a7b0-255e6263c9f7 (accessed 20 May 2021).

Cook, A. (2019) Taking a holistic approach to acute mental health crisis. *Journal of Paramedic Practice*, 11(10), 426–432.

CQC (Care Quality Commission) (2020) *Assessment of Mental Health Services in Acute Trusts*. Available at: https://www.cqc.org.uk/sites/default/files/20201016b_AMSAT_report.pdf (accessed 10 May 2021).

Dawson, J. and Szmukler, G. (2006) Fusion of mental health and incapacity legislation. *British Journal of Psychiatry*, 188, 504–509.

Department of Health and Social Care (2018) *Modernising the Mental Health Act.* Available at: https://assets.publishing.service.gov.uk/government/uploads/system/uploads/attachment_data/file/778897/Modernising_the_Mental_Health_Act_-_increasing_choice__reducing_compulsion.pdf (accessed 21 January 2021).

DH (Department of Health) (2015) *Department of Health Guidance: Response to the Supreme Court Judgment/Deprivation of Liberty Safeguards.* Available at: https://assets.publishing.service.gov.uk/government/uploads/system/uploads/attachment_data/file/485122/DH_Consolidated_Guidance.pdf (accessed 10 May 2021).

Duncan, E., Best, C., Dougall, N., Skar, S., Evans, J., Corfield, A., Fitzpatrick, D., Goldie, I., Maxwell, M., …. and Wojcik, W. (2019) Epidemiology of emergency ambulance service calls related to mental health problems and self harm: A national record linkage study. *Scandinavian Journal of Trauma, Resuscitation and Emergency Medicine.* Available at: https://sjtrem.biomedcentral.com/articles/10.1186/s13049-019-0611-9 (accessed 21 March 2021).

Eaton, G., Wong, G., Williams, V., Roberts, N. and Mahtani, K. (2020) Contribution of paramedics in primary and urgent care: A systematic review. *British Journal of General Practice.* Available at: https://bjgp.org/content/70/695/e421 (accessed 21 March 2021).

Health and Care Professions Council (2018) *Change to SET 1 for Paramedics.* Available at: https://www.hcpc-uk.org/education/resources/education-standards/changes-to-set-1-for-paramedics/ (accessed 21 March 2021).

HM Government (2011) No health without mental health. Available at: https://assets.publishing.service.gov.uk/government/uploads/system/uploads/attachment_data/file/138253/dh_124058.pdf (accessed 29 March 2021).

HM Government and Mind (2014) *The Crisis Care Concordat.* Available at: https://www.crisiscareconcordat.org.uk/ (accessed 23 March 2021).

Hub of Hope (2021) Hub of Hope – There's always someone to talk to. Available at: https://hubofhope.co.uk/ (accessed 21 April 2021).

Hughes, O. (2019) Paramedics to get access to mental health crisis plans. Available at: https://www.digitalhealth.net/2019/10/paramedics-to-get-access-to-mental-health-crisis-plans/ (accessed 19 April 2021).

Hutchison, T., Lees, C., Lotto, R., White, A. and Harris, R. (2019) Clinical decision making and the challenges of responding to mental health needs. *Journal of Paramedic Practice: The Clinical Monthly for Emergency Care Professionals*, 11(10), 434–439.

Jackson, E. (2018) From 'Doctor knows best' to dignity: Placing adults who lack capacity at the centre of decisions about their medical treatment. *Modern Law Review*, 81(2), 247–281.

Javed, A. and Herrman, H. (2017) Involving patients, carers, and families: An international perspective on emerging priorities. *British Journal of Psychiatry International*, 14(1), 1–4.

JRCALC (2021) *JRCALC Guidance.* Available at: https://www.jrcalc.org.uk/ (accessed 19 April 2021).

JRCALC and AACE (2019) *JRCALC Clinical Guidelines.* Bridgwater: Class Professional Publishing.

Keown, P., French, J., Gibson, G., Newton, E., Cull, S., Brown, P., Parry, J., Lyons, D. and McKinnon, I. (2016) Too much detention? Street Triage and detentions under Section 136 Mental Health Act in the North-East of England: A descriptive study of the effects of a Street Triage intervention. *British Medical Journal Open*. Available at: https://bmjopen.bmj.com/content/6/11/e011837.info (accessed 20 May 2021).

Lloyd-Evans, B., Lamb, D., Barnby, J., Eskinazi, M., Turner, A. and Johnson, S. (2018) Mental health crisis resolution teams and crisis care systems in England: A national survey. *British Journal of Psychiatry*, 42(4), 146–151.

Lovegrove, M. and Davis, J. (2013) *Paramedic Evidence-Based Education Project (PEEP) End of Study Report*. Available at: https://www.hee.nhs.uk/sites/default/files/documents/PEEP-Report.pdf (accessed 1 May 2021).

Mental Capacity Act (2005) Available at: https://www.legislation.gov.uk/ukpga/2005/9/contents (accessed 14 April 2021).

Mental Health Act (1983) Available at: https://www.legislation.gov.uk/ukpga/1983/20/contents (accessed 20 March 2021).

Mind (2020) Crisis services and planning. Available at: https://www.mind.org.uk/information-support/guides-to-support-and-services/crisis-services/ (accessed 2 April 2021).

Newton, A. (2012) The ambulance service: The past, present and future. *Journal of Paramedic Practice*, 4(5), 303–305.

NHS Digital (2019) National Record Locator for ambulance services. Available at: https://digital.nhs.uk/services/national-record-locator/national-record-locator-for-ambulance-services (accessed 12 April 2021).

NHS England (2015) Transforming urgent and emergency care services in England – Clinical Models for ambulance services. Available at: https://www.nhs.uk/nhsengland/keogh-review/documents/uecr-ambulance-guidance-fv.pdf (accessed 25 May 2021).

NHS England (2018) Commissioning framework: A framework for the commissioning of ambulance services. Available at: https://www.england.nhs.uk/wp-content/uploads/2018/09/commissioning-framework-and-national-urgent-and-emergency-ambulance-services-specification.pdf (accessed 3 June 2021).

NHS England (2021) Ambulance quality indicators data 2021–22. Available at: https://www.england.nhs.uk/statistics/statistical-work-areas/ambulance-quality-indicators/ambulance-quality-indicators-data-2021-22/ (accessed 25 May 2021).

NHS England and NHS Improvement (2020) *Mental Health Joint Response Car Pilot – Evaluation Report*. Available at: https://aace.org.uk/wp-content/uploads/2020/08/MHJRC-Review-Final-12082020.pdf (accessed 14 April 2021).

NICE (National Institute of Clinical Excellence) (2011) *Self-harm in Over 8s: Long-Term Management*. Available at: https://www.nice.org.uk/guidance/cg133/chapter/1-Guidance (accessed 2 May 2021).

Nuffield Trust (2020) *Ambulance Response Times*. Available at: https://www.nuffieldtrust.org.uk/resource/ambulance-response-times (accessed 27 March 2021).

O'Hara, R., Johnson, M., Niroshan Siriwardena, A., Weyman, A., Turner, J., Deborah, S., Mortimer, P., Newman, C., Hirst, E., … and Shewan, J. (2015) A qualitative study of systemic influences on paramedic decision making: Care transitions and patient safety. *Journal of Health Services Research and Policy*, 20(1), 45–53.

Pelto-Piri, V., Engstrom, K. and Engstrom, I. (2013) Paternalism, autonomy and reciprocity: Ethical perspectives in encounters with patients in psychiatric in-patient care. *BMC Medical Ethics*, 14(1), 1–8.

Policing and Crime Act (2017) Available at: https://www.legislation.gov.uk/ukpga/2017/3/contents (accessed 21 March 2021).

Prothero, L. and Cooke, P. (2016) Mental health crisis in the pre-hospital setting. *Emergency Medicine Journal*, 33(9), 1–2.

RCP (Royal College of Psychiatrists) (2020) *Self-harm and Suicide in Adults: Final Report of the Patient Safety Group.* Available at: https://www.rcpsych.ac.uk/docs/default-source/improving-care/better-mh-policy/college-reports/college-report-cr229-self-harm-and-suicide.pdf?sfvrsn=b6fdf395_10 (accessed 2 May 2021).

Rees, N., Porter, A., Rapport, F., Hughes, S. and John, A. (2018) Paramedics' perceptions of the care they provide to people who self-harm: A qualitative study using evolved grounded theory methodology. *PLoS One.* Available at: https://journals.plos.org/plosone/article?id=10.1371/journal.pone.0205813 (accessed 30 March 2021).

Rolfe, U., Pope, C. and Crouch, R. (2020) Paramedic performance when managing patients experiencing mental health issues: Exploring paramedics' presentation of self. *International Emergency Nursing.* Available at: https://www.sciencedirect.com/science/article/pii/S1755599X19301193?via%3Dihub#b0100 (accessed 27 March 2021).

Smith, R., Parent, A., Townsend, R. and Johnston, T. (2020) Mental health education in Australian paramedic curricula: A scoping review. *Australasian Journal of Paramedicine*, 17, 1–9.

Sondhi, A., Luger, L., Toleikyte, L. and Williams, E. (2018) Patient perspectives of being detained under Section 136 of the Mental Health Act: Findings from a qualitative study in London. *Medicine, Science and the Law*, 58(3), 159–167.

Thomas, K., Owino, H., Ansari, S., Adams, L., Cyr, J., Gaynes, B. and Glickman, S. (2019) Patient-centered values and experiences with emergency department and mental health crisis care. *Administration and Policy in Mental Health*, 45(4), 611–622.

6 The role of mental health social workers in crisis work

Values, responsibilities, powers and duties

Robert Lomax and Kevin Stone

In this chapter, we will explore the role that mental health social work plays in crisis work. Social workers work within legal and policy frameworks, with duties and powers they fulfil. Social workers will sometimes, through these frameworks, be able to offer help and solutions to crisis situations. On other occasions, the statutory imperative that influences many aspects of social work practice might limit their involvement. The nature and circumstances of a person's crisis are very relevant to how a social worker will be able to respond, especially if they are employed by a local authority. This chapter will discuss how social workers bring their own professional skills and capabilities to support service users, carers, and colleagues to resolve crises, and in doing so, determine their role within a multi-disciplinary and interprofessional health and social care context.

Introduction

Qualified social workers work in various health, social care, voluntary, and independent settings. Nationally and internationally, they work with individuals, groups and communities within society. Social workers in England and Wales must, by law, be registered with Social Work England (SWE) or Social Care Wales (SCW). The largest employers of social workers are local authorities who employ practitioners in children and families, adults, learning disabilities, and mental health teams. The last group is the focus of this chapter, as they are often working in a dedicated way to support people experiencing mental health difficulties. However, social workers in any setting may well be part of a multi-disciplinary or interprofessional team working with a family or individual. The majority of the time, mental health practitioners work in a supportive way fulfilling therapeutic and care management roles. In part though, these social workers remain agents of statutory control, playing a key role in the allocation of resources and through detaining and/or restricting the liberty of service users, as a consequence of assessments under the Mental Health Act (MHA) 1983 (2007), and/or the Deprivation of Liberty Safeguards, introduced as an amendment to the Capacity Act 2005.

Qualifying social work education programmes, registration with SWE or SCW, and optional professional membership with the British Association of Social Workers (BASW), if that is chosen, require social workers to affirm that they will, like other professions, practise ethically and in line with professional values. These values for social work will be discussed later. For now, it is enough to note that in terms of a bio-psycho-social holistic perspective, as to what contributes to and maintains poor mental health, social workers largely focus on the social and psychological aspects of that model. In this sense, social workers are focused more on the social determinants of health, and where change, adaptation, learning, or control are needed. The social perspective of mental health is distinctly different to the Social Model of Disability (Oliver, 1983) but both place an emphasis away from purely biological, pharmacological determinism, which can dominate mental health practice more generally. Social work draws most of its knowledge and approach from sociology and psychology, framed in a desire to achieve social justice, promote human rights, and empower, so that positive change can be realised.

This chapter will examine in greater detail the value that mental health social work brings to crisis work, and the roles that social workers occupy in this pursuit. First, the design of services where social workers are located is briefly reviewed. Then, the legislation, codes, policy, and guidance are noted, before a more in-depth consideration of the role in mental health social work is discussed.

Design of services

Mental health social workers work in a variety of settings, with approximately 5,000 practitioners employed within local authorities, and 2,500 employed or working within National Health Service (NHS) Trusts in England and Wales (NHS Benchmarking, 2020). A number of practitioners will also work in the voluntary, charity, and independent sectors. Social work services differ in their organisational design depending on a variety of factors. Most critical is the organisational relationship between the local authority and other organisations, principally the NHS, delivering local mental health services. Some social workers employed by the local authority will be members of multi-disciplinary teams based within NHS mental health trusts. Alternatively, they may be members of adult care local authority teams. Approved Mental Health Professional (AMHP) qualified social work practitioners may be located in either setting, but the managerial responsibility for their work under the MHA 1983 (2007) resides with the local authority.

Out-of-hours mental health services also vary in design and function. In some local authority areas, an Emergency Duty Team (EDT) service will operate. This service will be staffed solely by social workers who will respond to urgent requests for assistance for the full range of adult and childcare issues. This generic service design means that social workers are most likely to only be involved in mental health crises when a request for a Mental Health Act assessment is made. For most other mental health crises, the generic emergency duty service will rely on other, extended hours, mental health service provision, i.e. the Crisis Resolution and Home Treatment Team (CRHTT), to assist service users and carers. In other local authority areas dedicated to out-of-hours, AMHP-only services are provided, with practitioners often being physically co-located with local out-of-hours mental health services.

In terms of crisis work in mental healthcare, social workers may be involved in several ways:

- Social workers are often members of multi-disciplinary teams and, like their nursing and occupational therapy colleagues, will be care coordinators for the service users they work with. Depending on local arrangements, when known service users experience some form of mental health crisis, social workers will be involved in coordinating and delivering the appropriate response. This might be a direct intervention by the social worker and/or it might involve colleagues from other teams, professional disciplines, or services to support them.
- Social workers, especially those employed by local authorities (even if they are physically located within NHS Trusts), often have specific duties under the Care Act 2014 to undertake assessments of need for service users and carers, or respond to safeguarding assessments.
- Mental health social workers will often have undertaken further specialist training to become an AMHP. This role is discussed in some detail in this chapter. While the social worker, an AMHP, may only formally be on duty to undertake MHA assessments on a given day, their knowledge and expertise regarding the appropriateness of statutory intervention in a crisis will always inform their work.
- Mental health social workers, like their nursing colleagues, may have undertaken training to become Best Interest Assessors (BIAs) under the Capacity Act 2005. The extent to which this role is part of their daily working life within their teams will depend, among other factors, on how local adult care services are organised.

Legislation, codes, policy and guidance

Local authorities provide services where there is a legal duty of care to do so. In this sense, local authority professionals are the gatekeepers of the resources to establish if that duty of care threshold has been met. Initially, this may involve an assessment or determination as to whether the local authority is the correct agency to be responding. For some assessments that the local authority undertakes (such as under the Children Act 1989, or Care Act 2014), it must be determined whether that duty is engaged for other legislation, such as interventions arising from the MHA 1983; where there is a 'reason to think' (s. 13(1)) threshold which must be met before, for instance, a request for an MHA assessment would be accepted. Therefore, social workers are interpreting the legislation, codes of practice, policy, and guidance to determine where there is a duty to act, relevant to that particular department's role and function. This can cause tensions, often when these processes, and the possible limits to what local authorities can offer, are not understood. In the following sections of this chapter, we will consider these differing frameworks and the professional roles. Familiarisation of these will assist the referrer to understand the criteria being applied to determine if a service, resource, or intervention might be offered by the local authority.

Typically, the source of referrals can be:

- family and friends;
- general practitioners;
- the police;
- secondary mental health services such as CRHTT and Community Mental Health Teams (CMHTs);
- places of safety, health-based environments, police stations, and others.

Referrals will be triaged to establish if the person at the focus of the referral is consenting to an assessment, e.g. for a Care Act assessment, or if they have been deprived or restricted of their liberty, and require a statutory assessment under the MHA 1983 (2007), such as s. 136 or s. 5(2). Section 136 MHA is a power a constable can use to remove a person from any place (other than any house, flat or room where that person, or any other person, is living) to a place of safety if it appears to the constable that the person is suffering from a mental disorder and is in need of care or control in the interests of that person or for the protection of other persons. The purpose is to enable them to be kept at the place of safety for an assessment under the MHA to be convened within 24 hours (this can be extended for 12 hours if it would not be practicable for the assessment to be carried out before the end of the 24 hours). Section 5(2) MHA is a power a registered medical practitioner or approved clinician can use to detain an inpatient for up to 72 hours to enable an assessment under the MHA to be convened. Lastly, a person may need assessing for detention in hospital in the interests of their own health and safety, or for the protection of others.

Roles in mental health social work

The involvement of local authority mental health services (including social workers) arises for a multitude of reasons. For example, support and care

Figure 6.1 Roles of mental health social workers

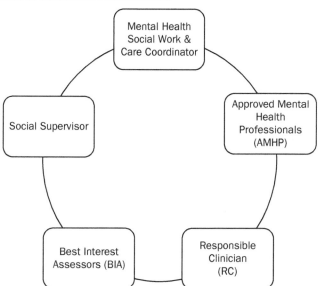

planning arising from Care Act 2014 assessments, where eligible mental health needs have been identified, or where signposting is needed to relevant community resources that do not require local authority involvement at all. Another area of practice relates to safeguarding adults. Although, as we have identified, the above design of services can differ, typically, mental health social workers are involved through a set of specific roles (Figure 6.1).

When engaging with a local authority for crisis work, some roles will be more readily visible than others, such as:

- Mental Health Social Workers – Care Act, 2014
- Care Coordinators – under Care Programme Approach (CPA)
- Approved Mental Health Professional (AMHP) – under the MHA 1983 (2007)
- Best Interest Assessor (BIA) – under the Deprivation of Liberty Safeguards/ Mental Capacity Act 2005.

These roles are considered below. Social workers may hold several of the roles as part of their employment, but undertake them to a different extent or frequency, depending on the tasks their employer requires them to undertake.

Mental Health Social Workers/Care Coordinators

Mental health social workers (MHSW) work with service users or carers in the community, as a care coordinator or a case manager, typically overseeing a package of care or support to enable a person's eligible needs to be met.

This may include duties under the Care Act 2014. As noted above, their location can differ, but which agency is involved will depend on which organisation has a legal duty to meet that assessed need. It is typical for post-registration social workers to begin their careers as care coordinators, before training for advanced roles such as AMHP and BIA. Mental health social workers may also engage in crisis work, through their roles in crisis teams and home treatment teams if they are employed by, or co-located with, NHS colleagues. The challenge here is for social workers to maintain their social care/social perspective, while working within a predominately medical environment.

The two advanced roles that mental health social workers undertake are practising as an AMHP and/or a BIA. Greater emphasis is placed in this chapter on these two roles, as their work is more frequently seen.

Approved Mental Health Professional: Mental Health Act work

Crisis scenario

Some events in people's mental health crisis escalate to a point where a person may need to be assessed under the MHA 1983 (2007) to determine if detention in hospital is needed. First, this might be if a person does not agree that it is appropriate for them to be admitted to hospital. Second, it might be if a person lacks the capacity, in relation to their care and treatment decisions, to agree to hospital admission when it is assessed by the appropriate doctors, and the AMHP, as being necessary. Equally, a person may be held to enable that assessment to occur, such as under s. 136 or s. 5(2) MHA 1983 (2007).

Background

Stone, Vicary and Spencer-Lane (2020) note that AMHPs are responsible for coordinating assessments under the MHA 1983 (2007), and for making the application for detention if needed. An identical power exists in law for a person's 'Nearest Relative' but, in practice, this is rarely used. Although the AMHP role can be undertaken by mental health professionals from other disciplines, social workers make up 95 per cent of the workforce (Skills for Care, 2021). When undertaking their duties, AMHPs may be located within their usual practice team setting, or may physically/organisationally move to an AMHP service located elsewhere. The AMHP service is sometimes located within a multi-disciplinary Crisis and Recovery Team, or might be a stand-alone service within the local authority.

When AMHPs are responding to a crisis by undertaking an MHA assessment, they must adhere to the provisions of the MHA and the guidance offered in the English Mental Health Act Code of Practice (2015) and the Mental Health Act Code of Practice for Wales (2016) respectively. The MHA Code of Practice (CoP) is a set of legal principles which must be followed, unless there are cogent reasons why adherence is not possible. These principles within the English code (MHA Code of Practice, 2015) are:

- *Least restrictive option and maximising independence*: Where it is possible to treat a patient safely and lawfully without detaining them under the Act, the patient should not be detained. Wherever possible, a patient's independence should be encouraged and supported, with a focus on promoting recovery wherever possible.
- *Empowerment and involvement*: Patients should be fully involved in decisions about care, support and treatment. The views of families, carers and others, if appropriate, should be fully considered when taking decisions. Where decisions are taken which are contradictory to views expressed, professionals should explain the reasons for this.
- *Respect and dignity*: Patients, their families and carers should be treated with respect and dignity, and listened to by professionals.
- *Purpose and effectiveness*: Decisions about care and treatment should be appropriate to the patient, with clear, therapeutic aims, promote recovery, and should be performed to current national guidelines and/or current, available, best-practice guidelines.
- *Efficiency and equity*: Providers, commissioners and other relevant organisations should work together to ensure that the quality of commissioning and provision of mental healthcare services are of high quality, and are given equal priority to physical health and social care services. All relevant services should work together to facilitate timely, safe and supportive discharge from detention (MHA Code of Practice, 2015).

The MHA and CoP are reminders of what Parliament intended, and how the judiciary have interpreted the provisions that Parliament set out. This means that there are limits to what an AMHP can legally achieve, and, also, due to the advanced training that they have received, why at times, those limits need to be reiterated to others who may feel that the MHA can be used (inappropriately) to find resolutions for a wide range of social ills.

Theoretically, a referral can arise from any source, although, in most cases referrers do not speak initially to an AMHP as front-of-house access is often staffed by administrators and call handlers. For an MHA assessment referral to be accepted, s. 13(1) needs to be considered:

> If a local social services authority have reason to think that an application for admission to hospital or a guardianship application may need to be made in respect of a patient within their area, they shall make arrangements for an approved mental health professional to consider the patient's case on their behalf.

The 'reason to think' trigger is an important one when coupled with the principle above, relating to 'Least restrictive option and maximising independence', as this means that undertaking an MHA should be the last possible resort, and not the first. There are situations when a person is detained to a place of safety under s. 136 by the police, or held in a place of safety under s. 135 following removal from a property, where some form of assessment under the MHA is unavoidable. However, requesting an MHA assessment should not be considered routine, and should certainly not replace a holistic mental health assessment undertaken by a crisis or home treatment, or psychiatric hospital liaison team. Therefore, although technically a referral for an MHA can arise from any person, unless the other alternatives can be discounted, a referral for an MHA assessment is likely to be declined.

The use of the MHA can be quite complex and the experience that service users are having can be distressing to work with. Consider the case of Amaka in case study 6.1.

Case study 6.1 Amaka

Trying to resolve Amaka's immediate situation has already involved the MHA and is likely to involve an AMHP warranted by the local authority, as well as NHS staff alongside other professionals. Central to how we treat people experiencing mental health crises is consideration of their fundamental human rights. The Articles of the European Convention on Human Rights (ECHR) (ECHR, 1950), the Convention on the Rights of Persons with Disabilities (CRPD) (CRPD, 2006), and other declarations or treaties need to be considered. As the ECHR Articles were given direct effect in UK domestic law, through the Human Rights Act 1998, these must be considered in everything the local authority and NHS do as a 'public authority'. At the referral stage, Article 8 ECHR, 'Right to respect for private and family life' subsections are important to consider:

1 Everyone has the right to respect for his private and family life, his home, and his correspondence.
2 There shall be no interference by a public authority with the exercise of this right except such as is in accordance with the law and is necessary in a democratic society in the interests of national security, public safety, or the economic well-being of the country, for the prevention of disorder or crime, for the protection of health or morals, or for the protection of the rights and freedoms of others.

(Article 8 ECHR, Human Rights Act 1998, Sch. 1)

For these reasons, the AMHPs need to understand fully what has been tried, why an intervention at primary and secondary care has not helped resolve the crisis, and what the risks are if an MHA is not convened – in this sense, justifying the 'interference'. There can be a concern at this stage, by AMHPs, that risks can be exaggerated, or not sufficiently determined, so that an MHA can be gained. Also, AMHPs will want to establish that any physical causes for the mental disorder presentation have been discounted. Therefore, there will usually be a discussion at the referral stage to ensure that an MHA is necessary, proportionate, and justified. Requests for MHA assessments, with the exception of s.136 referrals, are not procedural and need to be investigated, because any resulting assessment may be intrusive and an interference with a person's Article 8 rights.

There may be safeguarding concerns associated with a mental health crisis, which fall under the Care Act 2014 and, as such, all agencies involved should make a safeguarding referral. Professionals should not assume or rely on the actions of the AMHP, or the provisions of the MHA in and of itself, to be the safeguarding response.

Approved Mental Health Professional: mental health crisis breathing space

Crisis scenario

Some people's mental health crises are, in part, caused by or feature financial stress or debt. If a person in that situation is receiving mental health crisis treatment – not necessarily detention in hospital – then protection from enforcement action arising from debt creditors may be available.

Background

For people residing in England and Wales who need respite from debt, the Debt Respite Scheme (Breathing Space Moratorium and Mental Health Crisis Moratorium) (England and Wales) Regulations 2020 offer protection. This includes provisions to temporarily stop action intended to enforce the debt, or freezing charges or interest on their debt. To benefit from the mental health 'breathing space' scheme, an AMHP must certify that a person is receiving mental health crisis treatment, by submitting evidence to support a referral to a debt advice provider.

Best Interest Assessor under Deprivation of Liberty Safeguards

Crisis scenario

In some scenarios people are subject to restrictions, such as living in a lockdown, where they are not free to leave and are being constantly observed – or put in place – as those caring for them believe that they are acting to keep a person safe. In situations like these, in hospitals and in care settings, arrangements need to be assessed as to their legality, despite, perhaps, the best intentions – in most cases – of those implementing those restrictions.

Background

All professionals should be familiar with undertaking capacity assessments under the Mental Capacity Act (MCA) 2005, as this is a core part of all health and social care work, based upon the principles set out below, and the functional and diagnostic test. Our intention is not to discuss this here, but to focus upon the distinct role of the BIA. There needs to be a clear distinction made between the BIA role, and persons undertaking assessments under the MCA 2005, as no mental capacity test outcome can authorise a deprivation of liberty.

As set out in Hubbard and Stone (2018), deprivation of liberty assessments will involve a BIA, undertaking functions under the Deprivation of Liberty Safeguards, to determine if a person's freedoms should be restricted to the point where that person is deprived of their liberty. The BIA undertakes their work by completing an assessment of age, no refusals, and their best interests. The supervisory body (local authority) may also ask the BIA to undertake a mental capacity assessment, and an eligibility assessment, if the BIA-assessor is also an AMHP. These latter two assessments can be undertaken by a medical assessor (a doctor), who is s. 12-approved under the MHA, alongside the mental health assessors' mental health assessment. The purpose of the assessment is to establish if the care that is in place is necessary to prevent harm occurring to the individual, and is proportionate to the identified risk of harm occurring.

When a BIA is undertaking their assessments, as with anyone undertaking a MCA-assessment, the following principles apply for the purposes of this Act:

- A person must be assumed to have capacity unless it is established that they lack capacity.
- A person is not to be treated as unable to make a decision unless all practicable steps to help them to do so have been taken without success.
- A person is not to be treated as unable to make a decision merely because they make an unwise decision.
- An act done, or decision made, under this Act for or on behalf of a person who lacks capacity must be done, or made, in their best interests.
- Before the act is done, or the decision is made, regard must be had to whether the purpose for which it is needed can be as effectively achieved in a way that is less restrictive of the person's rights and freedom of action.

Case study 6.2 of Oisin provides an indication of some of the issues that a BIA might face in the course of their work.

Case study 6.2   Oisin

Oisin is a 19-year-old transgender male from Northern Ireland who has recently been involved in a serious life-changing motorbike accident resulting in a brain injury. The hospital staff are very concerned about Oisin as, although he has regained consciousness, he is trying to leave the ward and staff have stopped him as they feared for his safety as he presents in a confused state and has become sexually disinhibited resulting in sexual acts undertaken in public places. Although Oisin's presentation may improve, they fear they are now depriving him of his liberty and therefore contact the local authority for assistance.

Oisin's situation means that the hospital staff are seeking to clarify, through a Best Interest Assessment, the legal position regarding his continued admission to hospital. An assessment by the BIA will likely be the initial response from the local authority. The BIA role is largely undertaken by social workers, alongside their nursing, occupational therapy, and psychology colleagues. Any professional who is concerned that a person may be deprived of their liberty without authorisation would make a referral to the local authority, if the managing authority, i.e. the place where the person is living, will not do so.

Approved Clinician/Responsible Clinician

Crisis scenario

Some people who are subject to Community Treatment Orders (CTOs) – s. 17A MHA 1983 (2007) may need to be readmitted to a psychiatric hospital, due to a deterioration in their mental health. In this instance, their responsible clinician can initiate a recall of the patient to hospital and, if needed, revoke the CTO, thus placing the person under s. 3 once again. This negates AMHP involvement through setting up an MHA assessment, as the person to be recalled is already liable to be detained. No MHA assessment is needed.

Background

Since 2008, when the MHA 2007 was implemented, the psychiatry role of the Responsible Medical Officer (RMO) was superseded by a new role entitled Approved Clinician. This new role can be undertaken by registered social workers, mental health and learning disability nurses, occupational therapists, and practitioner psychologists once the competencies required for the approved clinician role have been met (DH, 2017), following engagement with the appropriate training (HEE, 2020). In these instances, the mental health social worker is employed by the NHS to fulfil this role. The uptake of this new role has not been significant, as largely it requires support from the NHS Trust employers. Thus, the majority of Approved Clinicians acting as Responsible Clinicians are in the main registered medical practitioners.

Social supervisor

Crisis scenario

Some people who are subject to a s. 37/41 MHA 1983 (2007) conditional discharge may need to be readmitted to a psychiatric hospital, due to a deterioration in their mental health. In this instance, it is the responsibility of the medical and social supervisor to contact the Ministry of Justice's Mental Health Casework section to discuss whether the person should be recalled. Although a person subject to s. 37/41 could be detained in hospital under s. 2 or s. 3 of the MHA 1983 (2007), this would need careful consideration. If they are held under s. 136, this would also need to be resolved first. The social supervisor is not necessarily a social worker, although they often are, and the medical supervisor is often their Responsible Clinician (see above).

Background

A s. 37/41 is a court sentencing disposal by a Crown Court judge, usually following conviction of a serious indictable offence, or a defence of 'insanity' has been accepted as a defence for murder. The s. 37 is a hospital order with a s. 41 restriction order, which is often referred to s. 37/41. If a mentally disordered offender is conditionally discharged by a tribunal (or by the Secretary of State), they remain on the s. 37/41, but are now conditionally discharged into the community. In these circumstances, the person subject to this order will have a medical and social supervisor appointed to oversee them. See also MAPPA below.

Responsibility for onward referrals

As with all professionals, mental health social workers have an equal responsibility for making referrals to involve other agencies – to safeguard and protect. This can often include making referrals to:

- Adult Safeguarding
- Children and Young People's Services
- Multi-Agency Public Protection Arrangements (MAPPA)
- Multi-Agency Risk Assessment Conference (MARAC).

All of these referrals will engage a multi-professional health and social care response, involving the local authority, and can include the involvement of the police. In some circumstances a direct referral to the police will be needed as lead agency.

Adult Safeguarding

Crisis scenario

In the course of your intervention, you become aware that a vulnerable adult with care and support needs is experiencing, or is at risk of, abuse or neglect and, as a result of those needs is unable to protect himself or herself against the abuse or neglect – or the risk of it (s. 42, Care Act 2014).

Background

A safeguarding adults referral can result in a s. 42 investigation, where the local authority must make inquiries or cause inquiries to be made. This work is undertaken in line with Chapter 14 of the Safeguarding of the Care and Support Guidance, issued under the Care Act 2014 (DH, 2014a). Here, it also outlines typical forms of abuse that professionals need to be aware of, but does not offer an exhaustive list, recognising that new forms of abuse arise as society's circumstances change and modernise. As set out in Spreadbury and Hubbard (2020), adult safeguarding is complex, but ultimately the purpose is: 'to promote and support the human and civil rights of adults who are unable to claim, and are sometimes prevented from claiming, their own rights' (p. 1).

One key consideration in this pursuit are agencies sharing information so that a fuller picture of a person's circumstances can be understood, and appropriate action taken (s. 45, Care Act 2014). Effective communication with the person on whom the concerns are focused is also key. As such, most agencies also have a safeguarding lead who should also be informed of the concerns. Local authorities will have a Safeguarding Adults Board (s. 43, Care Act 2014), whose purpose is 'to help and protect adults in its area in cases of the kind described in section 42(1)'.

Liaison with Children and Young People's Services

Crisis scenario

In the course of your practice, you become aware of a child in need and, as such, they are unlikely to achieve or maintain, or to have the opportunity of achieving or maintaining, a reasonable standard of health or development, without the provision for them of services by a local authority. Their health or development is likely to be significantly impaired, or further impaired, without the provision for them of such services; or they are disabled (s. 17 (10), Children Act 1989). Or, in more serious scenarios where you suspect a child may be suffering, or likely to suffer, significant harm. This includes child sexual exploitation.

Background

Contacting Children and Young People's Services is a key step in gaining support for a family, and, if significant harm is suspected, also gaining protective interventions through causing the local authority to make enquiries they consider necessary. This enables them to decide whether they should take any action to safeguard or promote the child's welfare (s. 47 (1), Children Act 1989). The role for professionals is to report concerns (sometimes immediately to the police) and inform the family that they are making a referral. This can often be a difficult decision for professionals to make, but it is important not to collude with parents, but support them to recognise that the child is the paramount consideration. This means that caution should be taken by not adopting wishful thinking, or embracing the rule of optimism by thinking everything will be resolved if a referral is not made. Or, worse, not referring because of an erroneous assumption that someone else will.

In the mental health context, placing emphasis on the protective aspect for an adult's mental health of having children, over the needs of the children's needs, must be avoided. Children being seen as a protective factor must not lead to that child not being brought to the attention of the local authority, or police in some instances. The needs of children must be given careful consideration in crisis work, given that children may be witnessing behaviours unusually uncharacteristic of their parents, or feeling sustained stress at needing to take on caring responsibilities beyond their age and maturity.

MAPPA

Crisis scenario

In the course of your work, a person who has been convicted of a sexual and/or serious offence, involving violence, may be referred to services. As such, under s. 325 (3) of the Criminal Justice Act 2003, professionals have a duty to work and cooperate with MAPPA responsible authorities, to manage the risk of eligible mentally disordered offenders (MHA 1983, Code of Practice, 22.87), meaning that you should liaise with the police, or other agency, if the presenting risks are evident.

Background

The purpose of MAPPA is to reduce reoffending. So, a crucial part of this work is identifying offenders, and enabling coordinated information sharing. Multi-agency public protection arrangements (MAPPAs) exist to assess, and then manage, the risks posed by sexual and/or violent offenders through the interventions of the police, probation, and prison services. The guidance (MAPPA, 2014, p. 1) states that:

> The Criminal Justice Act 2003 ('CJA 2003') provides for the establishment of Multi-Agency Public Protection Arrangements ('MAPPA') in each of the 42 criminal justice areas in England and Wales. These are designed to protect the public, including previous victims of crime, from serious harm by sexual and violent offenders. They require the local criminal justice agencies and other bodies dealing with offenders to work together in partnership in dealing with these offenders.

Identification of MAPPA-eligible offenders is the responsibility of each agency, including clinical commissioning groups and health trusts. A referral should be made to the single point of access; as agreed in each geographical area. This may be needed when an offender is subject to Level 1 monitoring, but new risk information suggests that this may need to be increased to Level 2 or 3 management. Referrals to MAPPA can be made by any Responsible Authority or Duty to Co-operate Agency.

MARAC

Crisis scenario

In scenarios where you are concerned that, as a result of domestic violence, there is a serious risk of harm – or worse, homicide – towards individuals or their families, a multi-agency approach will be needed.

Background

Although MARACs are not statutory bodies, local authorities can take a lead role. MARACs' primary focus is to safeguard an adult victim of domestic abuse. The MARAC process involves making a referral to a multi-agency conference to enable information to be shared about a victim of domestic abuse to professionals from criminal justice agencies, such as the police and probation, alongside health and social care agencies, including housing and specialist Independent Domestic Violence Advisors (IDVAs).

Collaboration with stakeholders: service users, significant others and other services

History and value of service user involvement in social work practice

Social work education and practice have always valued the contribution of people with lived experience of mental health issues. Their experiences, good or bad, have been important in informing the development of social work education and professional practice. Among other professions, social work has been praised for its progressive approach, especially in trying to include 'hard-to-reach' service user groups (Croisdale-Applby, 2014). The social work role has been interpreted by some as a partnership between service user and worker, with the practitioner supporting the service users to make change, working with them in their community, promoting preventive work, and enabling them to address the problems that they face (Asquith *et al.*, 2005).

Social work perspective and holistic assessment

Social work practitioners are trained to undertake holistic assessments of service users' circumstances. Professional training teaches practitioners the value of the Social Model of Disability (Oliver, 1983), and how the barriers that society creates can have the most negative impact on someone's day-to-day life. The difficulties that people experience are not necessarily, or solely, illnesses, conditions, or disabilities, that are located within the individual. A holistic assessment enables practitioners to appreciate that it is the wider cultural and structural factors, as well as personal ones, that may impact on an individual's health and welfare (Thompson, 2020). There has also been a renewed emphasis on practitioners recognising the role of poverty (Cummins, 2018) on the people they work with, and the role of other social determinants of mental health.

Social determinants of mental health

The social determinants of health are the 'conditions in which people are born, grow, live, work and age, and inequities in power, money and resources' (Marmot *et al.*, 2010, p. 16). This is the territory of social work, and this wider perspective on what contributes to crisis requires collaborative practice to help resolve crises.

The landmark study, *Fair Society, Healthy Lives: The Marmot Review* (2010), confirmed unequal societies are more unhealthy societies. A gradient of health was established, which indicated that all members of society (apart from those at the very 'top') had worse health than they might otherwise have had because of the inequalities in housing, income, education, and healthcare that exists in society. Marmot was clear that it is the social and economic circumstances of a community, a town, a city, that have the most influence on the level of health inequalities. Reduce the gradient of the curve, and everyone benefits. Health inequalities apply to mental health as well as physical health. The social determinants of health have been described as the causes of the causes.

The social work profession has long been aware of the impact of social factors on people's mental health (Bywaters, 2009). The Commission for Equality in Mental Health (2020) suggests that the inequalities in mental health can be framed in three dimensions: (1) social and economic determinants; (2) inequality of access to services; and (3) inequality of outcome of the experience of using services.

In terms of crisis work, an understanding of mental health inequalities, and the social determinants of mental health, offers practitioners a more nuanced and rounded appreciation of the context and circumstances that may have led to an individual's personal mental health crisis. Collaboration – in the widest sense of the word – with community resources and services to support service users in crisis, is vital.

The crisis might have its antecedents in the social determinants of mental health. We all embody our lived experience of the circumstances that have impacted on our health (Krieger, 2016), and the crisis in a person's mental health will result, in part, from the cumulative toll that the social, economic and environmental factors have had. Since the COVID-19 pandemic, the inequalities in society have been exposed afresh (Marmot, 2020a), and the role of social determinants in contributing to people's experiences is even more evident (Marmot, 2020b).

Collaborative working: professional sense or policy requirement?

Collaboration is a central tenet of professional mental health social work practice (Allen, 2014), and in mental health crises, its relevance is clear. As discussed, social workers practise in a number of different settings, and their ability to form good working relationships with other professionals is key. Collaboration involves the sharing of specific knowledge and skills to contribute to problem solving and crisis resolution. While legislation, such as the MHA 1983 (2007), and Care Act 2014, or policies such as the Crisis Care Concordat (DH, 2014b), make collaborative working a policy requirement, it is also a key aspect of good practice, as discussed below.

Social work good practice

Values

Mental health social workers, practising in the circumstances of service users' crises, should continue to adhere to, and enact, the values of the profession. The international definition of social work notes that it 'is a practice-based profession and an academic discipline that promotes social change and development, social cohesion, and the empowerment and liberation of people' (International Federation of Social Work, 2014, n.p.). At the profession's core is a concern for marginalised and oppressed groups within society. Many of the service users that practitioners have contact with will be from some of the most marginalised and oppressed groups in society, and a core concern for the profession is the welfare of those people.

Social work values are based on the respect for equality, worth and dignity of all people (BASW, 2014). Social work values refer to 'a range of beliefs about what is regarded as worthy or valuable in a social work context' (BASW, 2014, n.p.). This includes discussions about the principles social workers should follow in their work, and the desirable qualities of professional practitioners. There is no one specific list of values but the British Association of Social Work notes that they are embodied 'in the profession's national and international code of ethics' (BASW, 2014). They can be summarised as follows:

Human rights

Social workers, through their practice, should do the following:

- Uphold and promote human dignity and well-being.
- Respect service users' rights to self-determination, to make choices and to make decisions.
- Promote people's participation and involvement in services.
- Treat each person as a whole individual, who is part of a family, a community, and an environment.
- Focus on the strengths of individuals, groups, and communities to promote empowerment.

Social justice

Social workers, through their practice, should advocate for social justice by doing the following:

- Challenge discrimination on characteristics such as age, gender, sex or ethnicity.
- Recognise diversity through understanding individual, family, group and community differences.
- Distribute resources fairly and equitably.
- Work in solidarity with others to challenge social conditions that contribute to social exclusion and, in doing so, work towards an inclusive society.

Professional integrity

Social workers have a responsibility to do the following:

- Uphold the values and reputation of their profession.
- Be trustworthy.
- Maintain professional boundaries.
- Make considered, professional judgements.
- Be professionally accountable for their judgement(s) and actions.

All social workers in the UK must be registered with their respective professional regulator in England, Wales, Scotland, and Northern Ireland. Each regulator requires its registrants to follow a professional code of practice, each of which highlights the importance of values and ethics in professional practice.

Social workers in mental healthcare, who are AMHPs under the MHA 1983 (2007), must also ensure that the principles set out in the MHA Code of Practice (2015) are adhered to. The principles apply across the professional roles for people who engage with the Act, such as psychiatry and mental health nursing. In particular, the principles link well with the social work values, but also apply to other approved professionals, such as nurses, occupational therapists, and psychologists, who undertake the AMHP role.

Collaboration

Social work has a long tradition of multi-disciplinary and multi-agency working. Within mental healthcare, since the 1990s, social workers have often been members of multi-disciplinary teams working within NHS Trusts (Onyett and Campling, 2002). These experiences are not always straightforward. While valued by colleagues and service users, social workers have reported a relative 'invisibility', finding it difficult to define their role and expertise (Morriss, 2017). This is perhaps, in part, due to the generic nature of the Care Coordinator role

(Bailey and Liyanage, 2012) but nevertheless, social workers can contribute particular expertise. Colleagues from other disciplines report that social workers do the following:

- Apply a social model to their practice.
- Provide leadership and guidance for complex casework.
- Support practitioners to provide enhanced practice interventions (Abendstern, Hughes and Wilberforce, 2021).

Social work is often described as a values- and relationship-based profession (Turney, Ward and Ruch, 2016), and this focus is welcomed by colleagues and service users. For social workers not based in multi-disciplinary teams, the importance of collaborative working is not diminished. In some areas of the UK, social workers will be employed in local authority-led specialist or generic adult care teams, distinct from their NHS colleagues. Here, relationships between agencies and disciplines may be harder to engender, but it does mean that social workers are firmly rooted within local services. This gives them knowledge about, and access to, other services relevant to users and carers of mental health services; for example, knowledge about local statutory adult safeguarding services (Spreadbury and Hubbard, 2020). Similarly, some areas have standalone Approved Mental Health Act services, which sees AMHPs employed, managed and located within local authority services. Collaboration is a key aspect of statutory MHA work, and one aspect of the AMHP role is to mediate between different services (Leah, 2020), often developing long-lasting relationships with local general practitioners, psychiatrists, police and housing services.

Resilience, reflection and the role of supervision

Service users in crisis may be experiencing great hardship and adversity. Practitioners, too, may find responding to the needs generated by those crises stressful. Mental health social work is a stressful occupation (Evans *et al.*, 2006; Huxley *et al.*, 2005), especially with regard to undertaking statutory tasks (Evans *et al.*, 2005). Successful social work is predicated on relationship-based practice (Ruch, 2005), and this focus on relationships suggests there must be a concomitant focus on the impact of working with emotions as an aspect of practice (Winter *et al.*, 2019). It is therefore important for practitioners to consider how they can maintain their own resilience and well-being.

Resilience is a contested concept focused on, in some way, how practitioners can manage their own well-being to meet the challenges of professional practice. A straightforward definition of resilience is 'an adaptive state and personality trait' (Collins, 2007, p. 255) or that it denotes an individual's ability to 'bounce back' (Grant and Kinman, 2013, p. 357). Some authors emphasise the importance of individual characteristics, such as enthusiasm and hope, as being important to develop or have, to maintain a personal resilience (Grant and Kinman, 2013). Other authors emphasise the promotion of organisational

cultures and environments which promote their staff's well-being and resilience (Collins, 2017).

Reflective supervision is an established aspect of good social work practice
(Fook, 2004), and it is a significant contributor to developing practitioner resilience within organisations (Beddoe *et al.*, 2014). The function of supervision
varies between agencies, and some may emphasise caseload management, but
it is also the opportunity for reflective conversations that appears to promote
the development of resilience (Collins, 2017). Timely and focused supervision,
focusing, perhaps, on recent practice moments involving interventions at times
of service user crisis, is important in supporting practitioners. Supervision
enables practitioners to process their feelings about a particular practice
moment, to reflect on the impact of their own role and identity on their practice, and to be reminded or reassert the professional values that guide their
work. While many aspects of organisational working life are stressful, providing supervision is one intervention that employers can make, which can build
practitioners' resilience (Ravalier, 2019) and create conditions that support
practitioners to remain in role (Frost *et al.*, 2018).

Decision making

As noted above, social work practice is value-based, and this informs practitioners' decision making. Working with crises, whether undertaking statutory
mental health assessment or not, it is important that practitioners can articu-
late how they make decisions. For AMHPs, though, the need to be able to make
legally defensible decisions, regarding depriving service users of their civil lib-
erties, makes this need all the more necessary.

Whether a decision is a good one or not is often assessed by its outcome. In
crisis situations, the immediate outcome will usually involve an attempt to
reduce risks, but the longer-term assessment of whether the decisions taken
were the right ones is harder to evaluate. In the current context of mental
health practice, decision making is often exhorted to be recovery-based and to
promote individual responsibility for positive risk-taking. Involving taking calculated risks with service users and significant others, positive risk-taking
aims to promote quality of life, and may lead to mitigating life-threatening risks
like suicide (Reddington, 2017).

Social workers need to use their skills of critical reflection to inform their
approach to practice (Fook and Gardner, 2007). Equally, critical analysis of the
presenting issues is vital. Practice wisdom is the knowledge gained from practice, based on professional values and ethics, often in specific contexts. Linked
with critical reflection, practice wisdom accumulates through experience and
observation (Chu and Tsui, 2008). Social workers, like other professionals, will
have developed expertise in coping with decision making in crisis situations,
which includes incorporating a focus on their professional values, such as promoting self-determination, social justice and human rights.

An approach that supports social workers to do this is offered by
O'Sullivan's (2011) 'Sound Decision Making'. It is suggested that, rather than

evaluating decisions solely by outcome, the process of making decisions is also important, leading to the proposal of aspects of sound decision:

- being critically aware of the practice context;
- involving service users and carers to the highest level;
- working collaboratively with others;
- using knowledge, thinking clearly and managing emotions;
- framing decisions on situations in a clear and accurate way;
- analysing options and basing choices on reasoned analysis;
- making effective use of supervision.

Social workers and other professionals can use this framework in crisis situations to help them make sure that the decisions that they may be about to take – the longer-term outcome of which may be unclear – can be grounded in good practice principles. It is a practical approach to promoting recovery-based interventions that promote service users' views and rights.

Conclusion

Mental health crises can take many forms, and require differentiated responses from mental health professionals. Social workers, typically employed in local authorities, play their part in multi-professional and inter-agency settings, to help resolve difficulties that service users experience.

Social workers bring a value-base to their practice, explicitly predicated on autonomy, human rights, and challenging social injustice. Social workers also adopt a socially and psychologically informed understanding and response to mental health crises. This is not to discount the role of psychiatry and the medical model, but to acknowledge and balance the diverse ways in which mental health crises can be understood. In particular, the social work profession has an established tradition involving service users in the education of professionals, and the organisation of services.

The social determinants of mental health offer an understanding of the 'causes of the causes' of mental health crises and can inform the social work response. Social workers are often located in stand-alone services, or integrated NHS teams, with their multi-professional colleagues. Their crisis response, role and duties, in whichever setting, will fundamentally be determined by the legal and policy framework that informs the profession. This includes assessment and safeguarding responsibilities under the Care Act 2014. Most notably, though, many social workers will also have undertaken specialist training to undertake duties as an AMHP under the MHA 1983 (2007).

A mental health crisis that results in a statutory assessment under the MHA 1983 (2007) will, almost by definition, be a very significant moment in a service user's life. An AMHP, typically, but not exclusively, social work qualified,

following the values of the profession and the principles of the Code of
Practice, will work to resolve the crisis in a way that respects, and is informed
by, the views and wishes of the service user.

Further reading

- **AMHPs:**
  Stone, K., Vicary, S. and Spencer-Lane, T. (2020) *The Approved Mental
  Health Professional Practice Handbook*. Bristol: Policy Press.
- **Mental Capacity Act and Deprivation of Liberty Safeguards legal
  framework:**
  Hubbard, R. and Stone, K. (2018) *The Best Interests Assessor Practice
  Handbook*. Bristol: Policy Press.
- **Overview of mental health and social work:**
  Golightley, M. and Goemans, R. (2020) *Social Work and Mental Health*, 7th
  edn. Basingstoke: Learning Matters.
- **Sociological perspective of mental health:**
  Rogers, A. and Pilgrim, D. (2020) *A Sociology of Mental Health and Illness*,
  6th edn. London: Open University Press.

References

Abendstern, M., Hughes, J. and Wilberforce. M. (2021) Perceptions of the social worker
role in adult community mental health teams in England. *Qualitative Social Work*,
20(3), 1–19.

Allen, R. (2014) *The Role of the Social Worker in Adult Mental Health Services*. London:
The College of Social Work.

Asquith, S., Clark, C. and Waterhouse, L. (2005) *The Role of the Social Worker in the 21st
Century: A Literature Review*. Edinburgh: The Scottish Executive.

Bailey, D. and Liyanage, L. (2012) The role of the mental health social worker: Political
pawns in the reconfiguration of adult health and social care. *British Journal of Social
Work*, 42, 1113–1131.

Beddoe, L., Davys, A.M. and Adamson, C. (2014) 'Never trust anybody who says "I don't
need supervision"': Practitioners' beliefs about social worker resilience. *Practice*,
26(2), 113–130.

BASW (British Association of Social Workers) (2014) *The Code of Ethics for Social Work*.
Available at: https://www.basw.co.uk/about-basw/code-ethics (accessed 2 May 2021).

Bywaters, P. (2009) Tackling inequalities in health: A global challenge for social work.
British Journal of Social Work, 39, 353–367.

Care Act 2014. Available at: https://www.legislation.gov.uk/ukpga/2014/23/contents/
enacted (accessed 8 June 2021).

Children Act 1989. Available at: https://www.legislation.gov.uk/ukpga/1989/41/contents
(accessed 8 June 2021).

Collins, S. (2007) Social workers, resilience, positive emotions and optimism. *Practice*, 19(4), 255–269.

Collins, S. (2017) Social workers and resilience revisited. *Practice*, 29(2), 85–105.

Collins, S. (2017) SociChu, W.C.K. and Tsui, M. (2008) The nature of practice wisdom in social work revisited. *International Social Work*, 51(1), 47–54.

Commission for Equality in Mental Health (2020) *Mental Health for All? The Final Report of the Commission for Equality in Mental Health*. London: Centre for Mental Health.

Criminal Justice Act 2003. Available at: https://www.legislation.gov.uk/ukpga/2003/44/contents (accessed 8 June 2021).

Croisdale-Applby, D. (2014) *Re-visioning Social Work Education: An Independent Review*. London: Department of Health and Social Care.

CRPD (Convention on the Rights of Persons with Disabilities) (2006) Available at: https://www.un.org/development/desa/disabilities/convention-on-the-rights-of-persons-with-disabilities.html (accessed 8 June 2021).

Cummins, I. (2018) *Poverty, Inequality and Social Work*. Bristol: Policy Press.

Curtis, L. *et al.* (2009) The expected working life of a social worker. *British Journal of Social Work*, 40(5), 1628–1643.

Debt Respite Scheme (Breathing Space Moratorium and Mental Health Crisis Moratorium) (England and Wales) Regulations 2020. Available at: https://www.legislation.gov.uk/uksi/2020/1311/made (accessed 8 June 2021).

DH (Department of Health) (2014a) Care and Support Statutory Guidance Issued under the Care Act 2014. Available at: https://assets.publishing.service.gov.uk/government/uploads/system/uploads/attachment_data/file/315993/Care-Act-Guidance.pdf (accessed 2 February 2021).

DH (Department of Health) (2014b) *Mental Health Crisis Care Concordat: Improving Outcomes for People Experiencing Mental Health Crisis*. London: DH. Available at: https://s16878.pcdn.co/wp-content/uploads/2014/04/36353_Mental_Health_Crisis_accessible.pdf (accessed 7 March 2021).

DH (Department of Health) (2017) *Guidance for Seeking Approved Clinician Status Via the Portfolio Route*. Available at: https://assets.publishing.service.gov.uk/government/uploads/system/uploads/attachment_data/file/652073/Guidance_for_Seeking_Approved_Clinician_Status_via_the_Portfolio_Route.pdf (accessed 7 March 2021).

ECHR (European Convention on Human Rights) (1950) Available at: https://www.echr.coe.int/Documents/Convention_ENG.pdf (accessed 8 June 2021).

Evans, S., Huxley, P., Gately, C., Webber, M., Mears, A., Pajak, S., Medina, J., Kendall, T. and Katona, C. (2006) Mental health, burnout and job satisfaction among mental health social workers in England and Wales. *British Journal of Psychiatry*, 188, 75–80.

Evans, S., Huxley, P., Webber, M., Katona, C., Gately, C., Mears, A., Medina, J., Pajak, S. and Kendall, T. (2005) The impact of 'statutory duties' on mental health social workers in the UK. *Health and Social Care in the Community*, 13(2), 145–154.

Fook, J. (2004) Critical reflection and organisational learning and change: A case study. In N. Gould and M. Baldwin (eds) *Social Work, Critical Reflection and the Learning Organisation*. Aldershot: Ashgate Publishing, pp. 57–74.

Fook, J. and Gardner, J. (2007) *Practising Critical Reflection: A Resource Handbook*. Maidenhead: Open University Press.

Frost, L., Hojer, S., Campanini, A., Sicora, A. and Kullburg, K. (2018) Why do they stay? A study of resilient child protection workers in three European countries. *European Journal of Social Work*, 21(4), 485–497.

Grant, L. and Kinman, G. 2013. 'Bouncing back?' Personal representations of resilience of student and experienced social workers. *Practice*, 25(5), 349–366.

HEE (Health Education England) (2020) *Multi-Professional Approved/Responsible Clinician Implementation Guide*. Available from: https://www.hee.nhs.uk/sites/default/files/documents/Multi%20Professional%20Approved%20Responsible%20Clinician%20Implementation%20Guide.pdf (accessed 7 March 2021).

HMSO (2015) *Mental Health Act Code of Practice*. London: HMSO.

Hubbard, R. and Stone, K. (2018) *The Best Interests Assessor Practice Handbook*. Bristol: Policy Press.

Human Rights Act 1998. Available at: https://www.legislation.gov.uk/ukpga/1998/42/contents (accessed 8 June 2021).

Huxley, P., Evans, S., Gately, C., Webber, M., Mears, A., Pajak, S., Kendall, T., Medina, J. and Katona, C. (2005) Stress and pressures in mental health social work: The worker speaks. *British Journal of Social Work*, 35, 1063–1079.

International Federation of Social Work (2014) *Global Definition of the Social Work Profession*. Available at: https://www.ifsw.org/what-is-social-work/global-definition-of-social-work/ (accessed 2 May 2021).

Krieger, N. (2016) Living and dying at the crossroads: Racism, embodiment, and why theory is essential for a public health of consequence. *American Journal of Public Health*, 106(5), 832–833.

Leah, C. (2020) Approved mental health professionals: Jack of all trades? Hybrid professional roles within a mental health occupation. *Qualitative Social Work*, 19(5–6), 1–20.

MAPPA (2014) Multi-Agency Public Protection Arrangements (MAPPA): Statutory Guidance. Available at: https://www.gov.uk/government/publications/multi-agency-public-protection-arrangements-mappa-guidance (accessed 6 April 2021).

Marmot, M., Allen, J., Boyce, T., Goldblatt, P. and Morrison, J. (2020a) *Health Equity in England: The Marmot Review 10 Years On*. London: Institute of Health Equity.

Marmot, M., Allen, J., Goldblatt, P., Herd, E. and Morrison, J. (2020b) *Build Back Fairer: The COVID-19 Marmot Review: The Pandemic, Socioeconomic and Health Inequalities in England*. London: The Health Foundation/Institute of Health Equity.

Marmot, M., Atkinson, T., Bell, J., Black, C., Broadfoot, P., Cumberlege, J., Diamond, I., Gilmore, I., … and Mulgan, G. (2010) *Fair Society, Healthy Lives: The Marmot Review*. London: The Marmot Review.

Mental Capacity Act 2005. Available at: https://www.legislation.gov.uk/ukpga/2005/9/contents (accessed 8 June 2021).

Mental Health Act 1983. Available at: https://www.legislation.gov.uk/ukpga/1983/20/contents (accessed 8 June 2021).

Mental Health Act 2007. Available at: https://www.legislation.gov.uk/ukpga/2007/12/contents (accessed 8 June 2021).

Mental Health Act Code of Practice 2015. Available at: https://assets.publishing.service.gov.uk/government/uploads/system/uploads/attachment_data/file/435512/MHA_Code_of_Practice.PDF (accessed 8 June 2021).

Mental Health Act Code of Practice for Wales 2016. Available at: https://gov.wales/sites/default/files/publications/2019-03/mental-health-act-1983-code-of-practice-mental-health-act-1983-for-wales-review-revised-2016.pdf (accessed 8 June 2021).

Morriss, L. (2017) Being seconded to a mental health trust: The (in)visibility of mental health social work. *British Journal of Social Work*, 47, 1344–1360.

NHS Benchmarking (2020) National Workforce Stocktake of Mental Health Social Workers in NHS Trusts. Available at: https://www.hee.nhs.uk/sites/default/files/

documents/NHSBN%20NHS%20Social%20Worker%20Findings%20for%20HEE.pdf (accessed 7 May 2021).

Oliver, M. (1983) *Social Work with Disabled People*. Basingstoke: Palgrave Macmillan.

Onyett, S. and Campling, J. (2002) *Teamworking in Mental Health*. Basingstoke: Palgrave Macmillan.

O'Sullivan, T. (2011) *Decision Making in Social Work*, 2nd edn. Basingstoke: Palgrave Macmillan.

Ravalier, J.M. (2019) Psycho-social working conditions and stress in UK social workers, *British Journal of Social Work*, 49(2), 371–390.

Reddington, G. (2017) The case for positive risk-taking to promote recovery. *Mental Health Practice*, 20(7), 29–32.

Ruch, G. (2005) Relationship-based practice and reflective practice: Holistic approaches to contemporary child care social work, *Child and Family Social Work*, 10, 111–123.

Skills for Care (2021) *The Approved Mental Health Act Professional Workforce in the Adult Social Care Sector*. London: Department for Health and Social Care. Available at: https://www.skillsforcare.org.uk/adult-social-care-workforce-data/Workforce-intelligence/documents/AMHPs-Briefing.pdf (accessed 5 April 2021).

Spreadbury, K. and Hubbard, R. (2020) *The Adult Safeguarding Practice Handbook*. Bristol: Policy Press.

Stone, K., Vicary, S. and Spencer-Lane, T. (2020) *The Approved Mental Health Professional Practice Handbook*. Bristol: Policy Press.

Thompson, N. (2020) *Anti-Discriminatory Practice*, 5th edn. Basingstoke: Palgrave Macmillan.

Turney, D., Ward, A. and Ruch, G. (2016) *Relationship-Based Social Work: Getting to the Heart of the Profession*, 2nd edn. London: Jessica Kingsley.

Welsh Assembly Government (2016) *Mental Health Act Code of Practice for Wales*. Cardiff: Welsh Assembly Government.

Winter, K., Morrison, F., Cree, V., Ruch, G., Hadfield, M. and Hallett, S. (2019) Emotional labour in social workers' encounters with children and their families. *British Journal of Social Work*, 49(1), 217–233.

World Health Organisation (2014) *Social Determinants of Health*. Geneva: World Health Organisation.

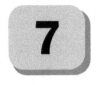

7 Collaboration and whole system working

Jo Williams and Kris Deering

The concluding chapter will draw on and collate themes from previous discussions across the preceding chapters and explore the vision of the Crisis Care Concordat which sets the standard for partnership working. This includes examining ways to work towards this goal, progressing from interpersonal collaboration to dovetailing provision, enabling the promotion of whole systems working.

Despite the different professional roles involved in crisis management, conceivably there is a shared ethic of helping an individual in distress. A focus will be placed on this notion and, even with differences, will recognise all helping professionals have a mutually shared aim to help. This will include an overview of the Department of Health (DH, 2004) ten essential shared capabilities: a framework for the whole of the mental health workforce, while outlining innovations that will help to build positive interactions between service providers with the aim of reducing emerging conflicts in the future.

To facilitate change means recognising and embracing potential opportunities and challenges and, as such, this chapter will explore barriers and enablers to restructuring services. Looking ahead, informing changes will require evidence of innovative ideas that will promote patient care and help develop interprofessional and collaborative working practices. Embracing innovative grassroots partnerships is key to reducing the challenges and stress caused to patients when seeking to access and navigate the complex terrain of services.

Introduction

As we approach this final chapter, it is helpful to revisit and draw upon the content of the preceding chapters in guiding us to situate our positionality, in relation to our learning and consider our actions about how we can move forward, and contribute to facilitating change in relation to supporting an individual experiencing a crisis. It is useful to pause, reflect and ask ourselves, what do I now *know* and, what do I now *think*?

What is evident throughout this text is that professionals currently work in 'silos' and often in isolation, either individually or as a service. The terrain of crisis support is complex and fragmented, and at times, because of this, impacts detrimentally on service users, leading to further distress and increased levels of risk (see mental health spectrum, Chapter 1).

We propose that to move forward and make impactful positive changes, adopting a whole system approach, whereby joined-up thinking and cross-percolation of ideas are used, is significantly pertinent. To help promote consideration of this, exploring the ten essential shared capabilities framework recognises that when a person presents in a crisis seeking help, the first 24 hours are key, thus helping to motivate interprofessional collaboration through a mutually shared vision.

Historically, the provision of psychiatric care has witnessed monumental changes, notably during the 1960s and furthermore, the 1990s, when the drivers of change sought to close large inpatient hospitals and redirect service users and their care, into the community. These closures were impactful across multiple strata in society (individuals, communities and nationally) but it is useful to recognise that this historical timeline is not time-limited; it is ongoing, hence moving forward progressively is fundamental to enable change. The text has been written by a diversity of professionals who have expressed calls for better interprofessional collaboration, suggesting a collective openness to exploring grassroots innovations, hence, these concepts will be further explored, starting with the whole system approach.

Whole system approach

System thinking is key to whole system working, considering the different systems involved to collectively operationalise crisis management (Stansfield, South and Mapplethorpe, 2020). Focus is on providing effective joined-up care that meets the needs of people experiencing a crisis to ensure coordinated planning and provision (Pomare et al., 2019). The changing landscape of service provision is not necessarily orchestrated by design, but influenced by the diversifying needs of society. The demand to transform can materialise rather unexpectedly, while systems rooted within original service establishments may encounter difficulties with adaptation (Cohen, 2017). As Chapter 4 (regarding the police) shows, conflicts can ensue, amidst the primary role of upholding law and order against the needs of those in crisis.

When large institutions were deployed to treat the mentally ill, particularly in the early twentieth century, the use of paramedics and police to provide care was perhaps unheard of. But through the policy of deinstitutionalisation, resulting with care provided in the community and the closure of large psychiatric hospitals, community services like the police, alongside healthcare, had to adjust (Bredewold, Hermus and Trappenburg, 2020). Despite developing new services like the Crisis Resolution Home Treatment Team (CRHTT) to aid community care, particularly when acute, with a view to reducing hospital admissions, it could be suggested that other services involved have been playing catch-up with the changing landscape of mental health needs. Even CRHTTs struggle with increasing demand, suggesting that, as a service, it too is not adapting quickly enough to meet the needs of society (Mind, 2021).

The critique above is not to pinpoint helping professionals resistant to change, rather it is to highlight how important it is that the services involved in crisis care are mapped out, and each role, or system, is understood to promote interprofessionalism and collaboration. All stakeholders, including service users and their loved ones, have an important role to voice concerns and identify methods to improve care, with the focus on promoting care that is more cohesive. This comes from an ethical position that the patient and their significant others are the focal point to work more together, not the reason divisive arguments occur over whose role it is to care in a crisis scenario.

Promoting collaboration is not something that happens well when a service requires something urgently of another. These moments, when emotions are potentially heightened and fear of blame might exist should an adverse incident occur, may turn into something akin to protectionism (King's Fund, 2018). That is, protecting oneself or the service from feeling unqualified to help, uncertain of how to navigate risks, and unsure what crisis management entails (Cummins, 2018). A number of arguments can be justified when stating with certainty that the role to assist is not a particular service's responsibility, but questions remain over how this serves the patient, for their needs will be unmet when such disagreements occur. Indeed, some arguments about appropriate service provider may take longer than the time needed to have supported the service user and their family (CQC, 2015).

For services to work towards a whole system approach, social connections are needed with others in order to understand different points of view of how issues emerge and seek ways forward (Winters, Magalhaes and Kinsella, 2015). This is the essence of whole system working. Of course, much intricate complexity exists, and numerous texts discuss how systems thinking is a complex and mathematical endeavour. It is further complicated perhaps by a sense of powerlessness to do something about it. While a concerted approach involving all stakeholders is an important way to mitigate issues, these can lead to unwieldy service improvement plans that have unintended consequences. Cohen (2017) suggests protectionism can rematerialise, seen with responses to complaints, galvanising further complaints out of attempt to mitigate, not by addressing the grievance, but by demonstrating the positive practices that do occur. Hence a one-size-fits-all reply, focused on organisational reputation, may perpetuate the very issues it aims to mitigate (Cohen, 2017).

Attempting to fix a whole system of mental health crisis care with a one-size-fits-all approach may lead to unintended wider systemic issues. This is something considered by complexity theory; this is a theory to understand complex patterns caused by the intersection of diverse moving parts, or services, with their own complex systems of helping professionals. Complexity theory considers the whole system, i.e. the different components of crisis management, and what emerges from its interacting parts, as such, it is a useful theory when looking at interprofessional conflict and crisis care (Long, McDermott and Meadows, 2018).

Complex systems are networks of people exchanging information and they favour the shortest optimal route, hence simple interventions are effective when making adaptions (Chandler *et al.*, 2016). Change can lead to unintended consequences, causing greater complexity, referred to as the butterfly effect, to symbolise the impact of ill-considered changes, even when small. A butterfly flapping its wings may influence air currents over one global location that eventually leads to a storm over another (Florczak, Poradzisz and Hampson, 2012). Systems work well when adaptive to external forces and when effective, manageable and practicable changes are contemplated to limit the impact of unknown side effects (Baxter *et al.*, 2018).

As will be discussed, the interactions of people are key to adapting systems, and as suggested by complexity theory, appear sometimes to have no hierarchical direction, but emerge out of values to improve care. Notable is the cultivation of triage services between police and mental health services, coming from grassroots innovation, not necessarily led by institutional or governmental drives (King's Fund, 2014). However, also recognised is the importance of reviewing centralised approaches, particularly commissioning. Broadly, the King's Fund (2019) proposes 'commissioning comprises a range of activities', including the following:

- assessing needs;
- planning services;
- procuring services;
- monitoring quality.

Local commissioning groups decide on the expenditure of resources, by offering contracts to those able to provide value for money. While such value is important, procurement can be based on old service designs split between health and mental health services, while commissioning of health services does not currently include social care and police (Rees, Miller and Buckingham, 2017). However, no single helping profession can, at this time, provide care exclusively and unaided to meet service user needs when in crisis (Winters, Magalhaes and Kinsella, 2015). Therefore, nationally, communication channels require commissioning across service boundaries to address the operational needs of crisis management (CQC, 2018). Social media can assist by using platforms like WhatsApp to share ideas and look at ways to navigate issues between services. But these tend to be innovations that arise through local services reaching out to each other to improve collaboration (Rolls *et al.*, 2016). Such strategies will be further discussed, underpinned by the ten essential shared capabilities for mental health (ESCMH), which is a framework for the whole of the mental health workforce (DH, 2004), with a focus on simplicity to promote interprofessionalism and collaboration, by revisiting expert by lived experience and personal recovery (see Chapter 1).

Simplicity is not the easiest and most convenient route; it involves manageable interventions to lessen the unknown consequences negatively affecting the operationalisation of crisis management (Kannampallil *et al.*, 2011). Hence achievable interventions are key to meeting the vision of the Crisis Concordat, improving interprofessionalism via promoting communication channels, and ensuring services work more cohesively when encountering a person experiencing a mental health crisis.

Ten essential shared capabilities

The text has considered numerous policies and reviewed the literature to outline the practices of helping professionals whom a person in a crisis will encounter within the first crucial 24 hours, however, questions remain as to what motivates collaboration and interprofessionalism. With fractures across services, issues of resourcing, and difficulties of mental health-related education, some stakeholders might be forgiven for having capitulated to an unwieldy system attempting to provide mental healthcare.

However, complexity theory shows that humans make systems and, essentially, to generate bridges across fractures requires social connectivity between stakeholders who have in common the goal of improving care (Baxter et al., 2018). As demonstrated in a recent literature review, values involve partnership building to enhance cohesion (such as co-production outlined in Chapter 1), to generate a 'third space' for developing shared ideas principally to cultivate communication channels and lessen conflict (Wranik et al., 2019). Rather than rely on institutions and/or government to make changes, although it is acknowledged that this is something that is required, it is the helping professionals, service users and their loved ones among others, who must collaborate to develop the interconnections required for whole system working (Wranik et al., 2019). Professionals reaching out require diplomacy, involving empathy and not blaming problems on other service providers. By doing so, dialogue moves beyond impasses and helps find a mutual ground within which to generate ideas to promote collaboration (Adamson et al., 2018; Turner and Baker, 2019).

While several readers of this text entered their professions to help others, a sense of fatigue has perhaps set in, feeling that the difficulties of crisis management are unsurmountable. In recognition that patients and significant others are the focal point of care, alongside perhaps a need to revitalise inspiration to work towards that goal, we recommend revisiting the ESCMH. Rather than an old government standard obscured by more recent policies, we propose the ESCMH is an ethical framework, that can inspire helping professionals to reach out to fellow service providers to promote cohesive and quality crisis care (Hope, 2008). The ESCMH will resonate with a number of helping practitioners to remind them why they entered their profession, as the capabilities act to resuscitate a vision of the importance of collaboration and interprofessionalism (Anderson and Burgess, 2009).

Argyris (1976) suggests analysis that examines the values behind the practice is likely to achieve sustainable and positive change. To an extent, this fits complexity theory, in that change to practices may only have unintended side effects, resulting in professional fatigue, not a desire to care more effectively (Lamb and Cogan, 2016). Technical abilities alone are perhaps superfluous without the drive to perform person-centred care (Anderson and Burgess, 2009). Moreover, grassroots consultation can be beneficial, as stakeholders who directly provide and/or receive care are attuned to the complexities of provision. The ESCMH is one such exercise, published in 2004, involving a large-scale consultation with service users and carers, mental healthcare practitioners and academics (Hope, 2008).

Service users and their significant others reported that a close, collaborative relationship built on mutual trust, respect and ethical practice is key to care, as such formed the basis of ESCMH values (Hope, 2008). Instead of being limited to those in receipt of care and their loved ones, attentiveness to ESCMH values is also required to be reciprocated among helping professionals to enhance practice (Brabban, McGonagle and Brooker, 2006). Accordingly, the capabilities illustrated below are an ethical force to motivate the generation of achievable changes with care provision and education, discussed further in the following sections.

The ten essential shared capabilities are:

1   Working in partnerships.
2   Respecting diversity.
3   Practising ethically.
4   Challenging inequality.
5   Promoting recovery.
6   Identifying the needs and strengths of people.
7   Providing service user-centred care.
8   Making a difference.
9   Promoting safety and positive risk taking.
10   Personal development and learning.

(DH, 2004)

Grassroots innovations

As previously mentioned, the UK has witnessed large-scale closures of psychiatric hospitals and notably, considerable changes to mental health provision, since the advent of the NHS (National Health Service) and the Community Care Act (1990). The Act brought about deinstitutionalisation, increasing community care for service users and shifting provision of mental healthcare, in particular, acute services that traditionally were reliant on hospital settings. This has not been without challenges. Davis (2006) and later Torrey (2010) are critical of the way deinstitutionalisation was operationalised, resulting in lack of patient support and increased substance use, homelessness, poor diet and nutrition, social isolation and worsening stigmatisation of individuals living with mental illness.

Fry *et al.* (2002) and Clarke *et al.* (2006) agree that hospital closures were a contributory factor in addition to the reduction and changes of service provision, meaning people who had previously been cared for in a hospital setting had limited personal resources and access to community-based services when they needed support. Hence, throughout this timeline, those experiencing a mental health crisis have felt they had limited choices and nowhere else to go, other than seeking help via emergency departments (EDs) and/or the police (the latter often being at the request of a service user's carer, relative or friend). Staff working in these settings/organisations often feel unprepared, ill equipped and lack confidence to help and support a person experiencing a crisis; the impact on the service user is that of feeling helpless, a burden, and not being prioritised, as a result.

What is evident throughout the previous chapters and supporting literature is the expressed calls to adopt and promote collaborative approaches to working with and supporting service users experiencing a crisis. Rossen, Bartlett and Herrick (2008) propose that interdisciplinary team working can present an array of challenges yet is immensely beneficial, not only for service users and their carers but also for professionals and other stakeholders. Craven and Bland (2006) sought to define collaborative care. They suggest that this involves a range of providers from across different disciplines, specialities and/or other sectors, who, by working together, ensure, where possible, a prompt response, appropriate care provided by the most appropriate person/professional/service and in a suitably convenient location.

Reeves *et al.* (2017) seek to define the terminology by proposing that interprofessional collaboration is where one or more health and/or social care professionals work together to improve their practice and they suggest there are three forms of interprofessional collaboration (IPC) explored further in the next section:

- Interprofessional Organisation (IPO)
- Interprofessional Practice (IPP)
- Interprofessional Education (IPE).

How can professionals collaborate?

Winters, Magalhaes and Kinsella (2015) propose four key actions for professionals to consider:

1 proactive and positive support for interprofessional collaboration;
2 improving care delivery systems;
3 merging distinct versions of care;
4 identifying and addressing emerging challenges.

Proactive and positive support for interprofessional collaboration involves identifying key services which are integral to supporting a person experiencing a crisis. For example, the professionals identified in this book but also others who could assist and complement the support provided by statutory services, notably the third sector with charities like Mind and Rethink (Machin *et al.*, 2019).

Care delivery systems can be improved by reducing/removing the burden for individual professionals within organisations. This is not without challenges; however, the complex nature of mental health crisis requires collaborative working with other professionals to ensure the care provided is beyond minimal, and results in positive outcomes for service users. Thoughtful acknowledgement and consideration of the uniqueness and diversity of individuality, of the patient, of their significant others as well as of fellow helping professionals, is essential to the provision and delivery of therapeutic care. As such, this underlines values adopted by the ESCMH for sustainable interprofessional collaboration.

Services espouse and employ differing models of care in their approach to supporting and managing a person presenting in a crisis. A number of services 'sit' within health and/or social care (e.g. CRHTT, ED, and paramedics), others 'sit' outside the health and social care system (e.g. police). Laing *et al.* (2012) suggest this can present issues and make IPC working challenging because of individual and/or organisational positionality and approaches when defining 'a mental health crisis'. The differing use of professional language and terminology should also be considered within the context of addressing improved care delivery systems (Dreher-Hummel *et al.*, 2021). This is because the use of specific language and terminology may significantly determine outcomes for service users, for example, 'healthcare provision versus public protection', and 'service user/patient versus detainee'. Key to addressing improved care delivery systems is recognising shared commitments to merging mutually agreed approaches (including the use of language and terminology) which reflect a shared vision and ethos of care for a person experiencing a crisis.

Acknowledging challenges exist and will occur is fundamental to making progress and achieving sustained changes to approaches. It is important to address issues such as lack of resources, time constraints, communication difficulties (including with service users and other professionals), lack of education training, and addressing stigma (across personal, professional and organisational levels) (Lackie and Tomblin Murphy, 2020). Collectively this involves changing the structures of services which work in a 'silo' format that result in professional isolation that is unhelpful for crisis care.

To change and reduce silo working, promoting effective dialogue is required, harnessing energy and collective motivation at grassroots level, among like-minded professionals, collaborating coherently, not just with other professionals but with service users and carers too. The aim is to review, evaluate and improve service provision, and triage care; consulting and talking with service users, carers, other professionals, and organisations, to cultivate communication channels. As proposed, attempting to promote partnership working is perhaps least productive when services are in urgent need of each other. Outside these times, meeting with other professionals can be beneficial if intention is to socially connect. By doing so, meetings are less intimidating, allowing opportunities to understand different points of view, and work towards solutions together (Maghsoudi, Cascón-Pereira and Beatriz Hernández Lara, 2020).

Interprofessional education

The concept of interprofessional education is aimed at promoting effective crisis management through interdisciplinary learning to enable the building of professional bonds (Reeves, Palaganas and Zierler, 2017). Like the Higher Education module that this text is based on, learning moves 'beyond the classroom', exploring innovative ways to promote cohesion across the fractured service provision that is tasked with supporting and managing persons experiencing a crisis. This involves ensuring the patient is central to the decision-making process, not the service/organisation, and being supportive of professional colleagues to work collaboratively alongside the service user (Winters, Magalhaes and Kinsella, 2015).

Ideally, interprofessional education can be achieved by involving all the disciplines discussed in this book and possibly others, who may complement their support. Such an approach to crisis management education enables professionals and other stakeholders working and supporting people experiencing a crisis to talk and meet with other professionals whom they might not usually meet (and work with), resulting in improved dialogue and reduced interprofessional/inter-service conflict (Broukhim *et al.*, 2019). Embracing grassroots innovation through productive dialogues represents a symbolic practice that is required to improve mental health crisis care. In addition, interprofessional crisis management education generates and promotes fertile foundations, creating cross-percolation of ideas and enabling professionals and stakeholders to explore and learn about the following:

- crisis management;
- collaboration;
- cohesive working practices;
- the creation of a shared space and effective co-production (see Chapter 1);
- the creation of an educational platform with other professionals on which to work and promote interprofessional management care;
- provision of balanced, equal representation and a contribution to local planning of crisis services.

The collective aim of grassroots innovations and interprofessional crisis education is to promote and ensure positive outcomes for service users and their significant others. As previously mentioned, this involves a tripartite co-productive approach (service user, family and/or friends and professionals), acknowledging that the service user is an expert by lived experience and through their experience of their personal journey of recovery (Church *et al.*, 2010). This includes understanding a broader range of service user needs, perhaps overlooked in crisis scenarios, such as social inequalities associated with mental health difficulties (Bergmans *et al.*, 2019).

The defragmentation of services seeks to enable better service user accessibility, but professionals may need to challenge the unconscious bias of others (professionals) as well as their own, for example, challenging negative stereotypes of fellow professionals that impact on abilities to collaborate. Giving due consideration to good ethical practice, as illustrated by the ESCMH, is key to improving crisis management approaches, be it in practice or in education, and goes some way to ensure crisis care service provision is therapeutic.

Conclusion

System-wide approaches to crisis management care can contribute significantly to reducing the silo-based working practices which have influenced the fragmented service provision that individuals and their families experience when seeking help and accessing mental healthcare in a crisis. However, as this text collectively demonstrates, the best practices of crisis care cannot work effectively without an integrated and connected system-wide approach which accounts for all stakeholders across the system.

Notably, recurring themes evident across the text include the role and value of co-production; ensuring a tripartite approach to crisis management care where service user and carer voices are encouraged and heard, giving voice to those often silenced. If we encourage and promote service user involvement, this will contribute to more open and shared dialogue, not only between professionals and individuals in their care, but between professionals and services/organisations, thus truly embracing the expert by lived experience concept.

When supporting an individual experiencing a crisis, professionals and stakeholders need to be aware and recognise the concept of recovery. As previously mentioned, when discussing the ten essential shared capabilities framework, the initial 24-hour period is key, and while arguably not viewed by the individual experiencing a crisis as part of recovery, it is a co-productive opportunity to support reconvening and re-establishing their perceptions of their own recovery journey.

Defining terminology and adopting a mutually shared 'language' is relevant to promoting the success of interprofessional collaboration. Differing interpretations of terminology (for example, crisis) exist, and this contributes to fragmented working practices whereby mutual understanding is not shared, leading to distorted perceptions and dichotomous approaches, which are unhelpful in supporting individuals in need.

Advocating and lobbying for interprofessional education helps create learning platforms with other professionals on which to share ideas, create a forum for discussion/debate and promote collaborative crisis management care. Where possible, professionals should contribute to planning local crisis services. This may include significant restructuring of what is already in existence or changing the spectrum of provision. By ensuring a range of crisis support services exist, and enabling the migration of services to a position prioritising the individual lived experience over the statutory risk-based frameworks currently dominating crisis care, this will create a shift in the gatekeeping power dynamic and promote more open, transparent dialogue and cohesive, collaborative working practices.

Further reading

- **Complexity theory:**
  Johnson, N.F. (2011) *Simply Complexity: A Clear Guide to Complexity Theory*. Oxford: Oneworld.
- **Expert by experience:**
  Basset, T. and Stickley, T. (2010) *Voices of Experience: Narratives of Mental Health Survivors*. Chichester: Wiley.
- **Interprofessional education:**
  Barr, H. and UK Centre for the Advancement of Interprofessional Education (2005) *Effective Interprofessional Education: Argument, Assumption and Evidence*. Oxford: Blackwell.
- **Interprofessionalism:**
  Reeves. S. (2010) *Interprofessional Teamwork for Health and Social Care*. Oxford: Wiley-Blackwell.
- **Whole system approach:**
  Peate, I. (2007) Mental health provision: Time for a whole system approach. *British Journal of School Nursing*, 12(10), 494–497.

References

Adamson, K., Loomis, C., Cadell, S. and Verweel, L.C. (2018) Interprofessional empathy: A four-stage model for a new understanding of teamwork. *Journal of Interprofessional Care*, 32(6), 752–761.

Anderson, J. and Burgess, H. (2009) Essential shared capabilities for the whole of the mental health workforce: Bringing the educators into the frame. *The Journal of Mental Health Training, Education, and Practice*, 4(3), 21–29.

Argyris, C. (1976) *Increasing Leadership Effectiveness*. London: John Wiley.

Baxter, S., Johnson, M., Chambers, D., Sutton, A., Goyder, E. and Booth, A. (2018) The effects of integrated care: A systematic review of UK and international evidence. *BMC Health Services Research*, 18(1), 1–13.

Bergmans, Y., Ninkovic, D., Sunderji, N. and Simpson-Barrette, D. (2019) Client evaluation of an interprofessional urgent mental health care program. *Journal of Psychosocial Nursing and Mental Health Services*, 57(3), 17–24.

Brabban, A., McGonagle, I. and Brooker, C. (2006) The 10 Essential Shared Capabilities: A framework for mental health practice. *The Journal of Mental Health Training, Education, and Practice*, 1(3), 4–15.

Bredewold, F.H., Hermus, M.M.J. and Trappenburg, M.J. (2020) Living in the community, the pros and cons: A systematic literature review of the impact of deinstitutionalisation on people with intellectual and psychiatric disabilities. *Journal of Social Work*, 20(1), 83–116.

Broukhim, M., Yuen, F., McDermott, H., Miller, K., Merrill, L., Kennedy, R. and Wilkes, M. (2019) Interprofessional conflict and conflict management in an educational setting. *Medical Teacher*, 41(4), 408–416.

Chandler, J., Rycroft-Malone, J., Hawkes, C. and Noyes, J. (2016) Application of simplified Complexity Theory concepts for healthcare social systems to explain the implementation of evidence into practice. *Journal of Advanced Nursing*, 72(2), 461–480.

Church, E.A., Heath, O.J., Curran, V.R., Bethune, C., Callanan, T.S. and Cornish, P.A. (2010) Rural professionals' perceptions of interprofessional continuing education in mental health. *Health and Social Care in the Community*, 18(4), 433–443.

Clarke, D.E., Brown, A., Hughes, L. and Motluk, L. (2006) Education to improve the triage of mental health patients in general hospital emergency departments. *Accident & Emergency Nursing*, 14, 210–218.

Cohen, M. (2017) A systemic approach to understanding mental health and services. *Social Science and Medicine*, 191, 1–8.

CQC (Care Quality Commission) (2015) Right here, right now: People's experiences of help, care and support during a mental health crisis. Available at: https://www.cqc.org.uk/sites/default/files/20150630_righthere_mhcrisiscare_full.pdf (accessed 22 June 2021).

CQC (Care Quality Commission) (2018) *Joint Framework: Commissioning and Regulating Together*. Available at: https://www.cqc.org.uk/sites/default/files/20180108_CQC_NHSE_NHSCC_joint_working_framework.pdf (accessed 22 June 2021).

Craven, M.A. and Bland, R. (2006) Better practices in collaborative mental health care: An analysis of the evidence base. *Canadian Journal of Psychiatry*, 51(6), 1–74.

Cummins, I. (2018) The impact of austerity on mental health service provision: A UK perspective. *Journal of Environmental Studies and Public Health*. Available at: https://www.ncbi.nlm.nih.gov/pmc/articles/PMC6025145/ (accessed 22 June 2021).

Davis, S. (2006) *Community Mental Health in Canada: Policy, Theory and Practice*. Vancouver: UBC Press.

DH (Department of Health) (2004) *The Ten Essential Shared Capabilities: A Framework for the Whole Health and Social Care Workforce*. London: Department of Health.

Dreher-Hummel, T., Nickel, C.H., Nicca, D. and Grossmann, F.F. (2021) The challenge of interprofessional collaboration in emergency department team triage: An interpretive description. *Journal of Advanced Nursing*, 77(3), 1368–1378.

Florczak, K., Poradzisz, M. and Hampson, S. (2012) Nursing in a complex world: A case for grand theory. *Nursing Science Quarterly*, 25(4), 307–312.

Fry, A.J., O'Riordan, D.P. and Geanellos, R. (2002) Social control agents or front-line carers for people with mental health problems: Police and mental health services in Sydney, Australia. *Health and Social Care in the Community*, 10(4), 277–286.

Hope, R. (2008) The Ten Essential Shared Capabilities: Their background, development and implementation. In T. Stickley and T. Basset (eds) *Learning about Mental Health Practice*. Chichester: John Wiley, pp. 7–21.

Kannampallil, T.G., Schauer, G.F., Cohen, T. and Patel, V.L. (2011) Considering complexity in healthcare systems. *Journal of Biomedical Informatics*, 44(6), 943–947.

King's Fund (2014) *Service Transformation: Lessons from Mental Health*. Available at: https://www.kingsfund.org.uk/publications/service-transformation (accessed 26 June 2021).

King's Fund (2018) *Making Sense of Integrated Care Systems, Integrated Care Partnerships and Accountable Care Organisations in the NHS in England.* Available at: https://www.kingsfund.org.uk/publications/making-sense-integrated-care-systems (accessed 22 June 2021).

King's Fund (2019) *What Is Commissioning and How Is It Changing?* Available at https://www.kingsfund.org.uk/publications/what-commissioning-and-how-it-changing (accessed 22 June 2021).

Lackie, K. and Tomblin Murphy, G. (2020) The impact of interprofessional collaboration on productivity: Important considerations in health human resources planning. *Journal of Interprofessional Education and Practice*, 21, 1–8.

Laing, L., Irwin, J. and Toivonen, C. (2012) Across the divide: Using research to enhance collaboration between mental health and domestic violence services. *Australian Social Work*, 65, 120–135.

Lamb, D. and Cogan, N. (2016) Coping with work-related stressors and building resilience in mental health workers: A comparative focus group study using interpretative phenomenological analysis. *Journal of Occupational and Organizational Psychology*, 89(3), 474–492.

Long, K.M., McDermott, F. and Meadows, G.N. (2018) Being pragmatic about healthcare complexity: Our experiences applying complexity theory and pragmatism to health services research. *BMC Medicine*, 16(1), 1–9.

Machin, K., Thompson, S., Poursanidou, K. and Moran, B. (2019) *Evaluation of Service User and Carer Involvement in the NIHR Funded Research Study: The Contribution of the Voluntary Sector to the Mental Health Crisis Care in England: A Mixed Methods Study.* Available at: https://www.birmingham.ac.uk/documents/college-social-sciences/social-policy/publications/involvement-in-crisis-care-study-final-accessible.pdf (accessed 29 June 2021).

Maghsoudi, T., Cascón-Pereira, R. and Beatriz Hernández Lara, A. (2020) The role of collaborative healthcare in improving social sustainability: A conceptual framework, *Sustainability*, 12(8), 3195.

Mind (2021) *Mental Health Crisis Care Services 'Under-Resourced, Understaffed and Overstretched'.* Available at: https://www.mind.org.uk/news-campaigns/news/mental-health-crisis-care-services-under-resourced-understaffed-and-overstretched/ (accessed 26 June 2021).

Mischen, P.A. and Jackson, S.K. (2008) Connecting the dots: Applying complexity theory, knowledge management and social networks analysis to policy implementation. *Public Administration Quarterly*, 32(3), 314–338.

National Health Service and Community Care Act (1990) Available at: https://www.legislation.gov.uk/ukpga/1990/19/contents (accessed 26 June 2021).

Pomare, C., Long, J.C., Ellis, L.A., Churruca, K. and Braithwaite, J. (2019) Interprofessional collaboration in mental health settings: A social network analysis. *Journal of Interprofessional Care*. Available at https://www-tandfonline-com.ezproxy.uwe.ac.uk/doi/epub/10.1080/13561820.2018.1544550?needAccess=trueand (accessed 22 June 2021).

Rees, J., Miller, R. and Buckingham, H. (2017) Commission incomplete: Exploring the new model for purchasing public services from the third sector. *Journal of Social Policy*, 46(1), 175–194.

Reeves, S., Palaganas, J. and Zierler, B. (2017) An updated synthesis of review evidence of interprofessional education. *Journal of Allied Health*, 46(1), 56–61.

Reeves, S., Pelone, F., Harrison, R., Goldman, J. and Zwarenstein, M. (2017) Interprofessional collaboration to improve professional practice and healthcare outcomes. *Cochrane Database of Systematic Reviews*, 6, 1–40.

Rolls, K., Hansen, M., Jackson, D. and Elliott, D. (2016) How health care professionals use social media to create virtual communities: An integrative review. *Journal of Medical Internet Research*. Available at: https://www.jmir.org/2016/6/e166/ (accessed 22 June 2021).

Rossen, E.K., Bartlett, R. and Herrick, C.A. (2008) Interdisciplinary collaboration: The need to revisit. *Issues in Mental Health Nursing*, 29(4), 387–396.

Stansfield, J., South, J. and Mapplethorpe, T. (2020) What are the elements of a whole system approach to community-centred public health? A qualitative study with public health leaders in England's local authority areas. *BMJ Open*. Available at: https://bmjopen.bmj.com/content/10/8/e036044.info (accessed 22 June 2021).

Torrey, E.F. (2010) Documenting the failure of deinstitutionalization. *Psychiatry*, 73(2), 122–124.

Turner, J.R. and Baker, R.M. (2019) Complexity theory: An overview with potential applications for the social sciences. *Systems*, 7(1), 1–22.

Winters, S., Magalhaes, L. and Kinsella, E.A. (2015) Interprofessional collaboration in mental health crisis response systems: A scoping review. *Disability and Rehabilitation*, 37(23), 2212–2224.

Wranik, W.D., Price, S., Haydt, S.M., Edwards, J., Hatfield, K., Weir, J. and Doria, N. (2019) Implications of interprofessional primary care team characteristics for health services and patient health outcomes: A systematic review with narrative synthesis. *Health Policy*, 123(6), 550–563.

Glossary

Acquired ability (to enact suicide) – Habituation to the thought of completed suicide, often explained because of exposure to various forms of harm, for example, combat or a history of self-harm.

Actuarial risk factors – Those factors that are deemed to statistically increase the likelihood of harm occurring.

Approved Clinician/Responsible Clinician (previously called Responsible Medical Officer) – An eligible and qualified professional who is responsible for the inpatient care of informal, voluntary, and involuntary patients.

Approved Mental Health Professional (AMHP) – An eligible and qualified professional approved under s. 114 Mental Health Act 1983 (2007) to make applications for involuntary detention to psychiatric hospital of persons who meet the criteria.

Best Interest Assessor (BIA) – An eligible and qualified professional who can undertake assessments under the Deprivation of Liberty Safeguards.

Bio-psychosocial perspective – A holistic perspective that is conscious of the biological, psychological and social context of a person.

Carer – An informal carer (family or otherwise) who provides a person with care.

Catatonia – A neuropsychiatric presentation characterised by a marked alteration in responsiveness to external stimuli, and abnormal motor function.

Clinical recovery – Care drawing on the expertise of clinicians about treatment options.

Closed questions – Questions that are likely to elicit a 'yes' or 'no' response.

Cognitive impairment – Deficits in cognitive functioning, for example, memory and attention span.

Collaboration – Many ways people can work more together to ensure all voices are heard whenever possible and that relevant stakeholders have a say in crisis care.

Common law – The part of English law that is derived from custom and judicial precedents.

Crisis Resolution Home Treatment Team – A health-based team that responds to mental health crisis to avoid admission to psychiatric hospitals.

Delirium – An acute and transient confusional state, precipitated by a physical trigger (e.g. infection, pain, constipation) and characterised by altered cognition, conscious level, and broader mental function.

Delusion – A fixed false belief that is not amenable to appeals to reason or logic and is out of keeping with the person's social, cultural, and religious background.

Deprivation of Liberty Safeguards – Contained within the Mental Capacity Act 2005, the safeguards authorise a person to be deprived of their liberty when the right criteria are met, and when the Mental Health Act 1983 cannot or may not be used.

Diagnostic overshadowing – The assumption by clinicians that a patient's symptoms are part of a mental disorder or pre-existing disability without exploring other possibilities.

Emergency Duty Team – An out-of-hours social work team usually containing Approved Mental Health Professionals and social workers from other disciplines.

Emotionally Unstable Personality Disorder (EUPD) – A long-term condition, characterised by an unstable sense of self, unstable relationships, and impulsive behaviour, including self-harm.

Empathic reflection – The skill of communicating back to clients that their thoughts and feelings have been understood.

Engagement – The process of forming a therapeutic relationship.

Expert by experience – Expertise drawing on the lived experiences of mental health and mental health difficulties.

Flight of ideas – A nearly continuous flow of accelerated speech with sudden changes from topic to topic.

Functional cause – Signs and symptoms that cannot be explained by observable structural pathology.

Hallucination – False perception without external stimuli.

Interprofessionalism – Whereby more than one professional works with another to meet a goal such as service user care.

Mental capacity – The ability to make a specific decision at a specific time.

Mental Capacity Act – Legislation designed to protect and empower people who lack the mental capacity to make decisions.

Mental disorder – A clinically significant behavioural or psychological syndrome or pattern that occurs in an individual and that is associated with present distress.

Mental distress – A range of symptoms experienced by a person that are commonly held to be troubling, confusing or out of the ordinary.

Mental Health Act 1983 – A piece of legislation that is used to respond to mental health crisis circumstances where all other options have not been successful.

Mental Health Act assessment – An assessment conducted by two doctors and an Approved Mental Health Professional (AMHP) to determine if an individual requires detention under the Mental Health Act.

Mental State Examination (MSE) – A formal structured description of a person's mental state as perceived by the clinician. This includes a description of the individual's appearance, behaviour, speech, mood, thoughts, perceptions, cognition, and insight.

Multi-agency working – Where practitioners from more than one agency/organisation work together, jointly sharing aims, information, tasks and responsibilities in order to intervene early to prevent problems arising which may impact on a person's mental health and well-being.

Open questions – Questions that are likely to elicit a fuller response (in contrast to closed questions).

Organic cause – Signs and symptoms that can be explained by observable structural pathology, for example, a brain tumour.

Persecutory ideas – Beliefs that other people are against an individual that often generate a sense of mistrust and suspicion.

Personal recovery – What service users and their significant others consider will be beneficial to develop a life that is meaningful.

Place of safety – A place defined by s. 135 Mental Health Act 1983 (2007) where a person can be removed to and kept for a Mental Health Act assessment to be undertaken.

Prevention and Management of Violence and Aggression (PMVA) – Formal training to reduce the risks of violence and aggression.

Protective factors – Those factors that mitigate against certain risks, for example, suicide or violence.

Psychiatric Liaison Accreditation Network (PLAN) – A network of liaison mental health services designed to facilitate improved quality and development in the field of liaison psychiatry.

Psychosis – A broad term associated with loss of contact with reality. In some cases, this includes the presence of delusions and hallucinations.

Psychosocial assessment – A comprehensive evaluation of a person's functioning including their psychological and social resources and areas of need.

Rapid tranquillisation – The use of medication by parenteral route for the purposes of urgent sedation.

Recovery – A focus on developing a meaningful life regardless of mental health difficulties.

Risk (concept) – Estimating the likelihood of a phenomenon through benefits and/or costs.

Risk (psychiatry) – Tends to be calculable harms that patients might inflict on themselves and others due to mental health difficulties, notably self-harm, suicide, and violence

Risk assessment – The process of evaluating the probability of harm occurring.

Risk management – Diverse combinations of decision making and interventions to lessen risk like suicide.

Service user – An alternative to the term 'patient'.

Shared decision making – A collaborative process involving the service user, health-care professionals and other key stakeholders to formulate a decision together.

Significant other – A person seen as significant to another, e.g. friend, family, partner to the patient as defined as someone of importance to them.

Somatoform disorders – A group of psychological disorders in which the person's symptoms cannot be fully explained by observable structural pathology.

Splitting – The failure to bring together the positive and negative qualities of the self and others into a cohesive, realistic whole. Splitting is sometimes used to refer to the process whereby people crudely divide others into 'good' and 'bad' categories.

Suicidal ideation – When an individual is having thoughts or ideas about ending their life.

Thwarted belonging – A risk factor for suicide in which the individual believes their connection with others is fundamentally diminished.

Thwarted effectiveness – A risk factor for suicide in which the individual believes that they have become a burden to others.

Voice hearing – The experience of hearing a voice when no one else is present.

Whole system approach – Involving ways that multiple systems, e.g. services, can work as a cohesive whole to meet some need, such as service user care.

Index

Page numbers in italics are figures; with 't' are tables; with 'b' are boxes; with 'g' are glossary terms.